Kate Carbery is a proud mother of two small children. An honours graduate of University College Cork, she worked in human resources and communications before setting up a medical company in Dublin with her husband. Kate has travelled extensively and studied and worked overseas. A natural storyteller, she has an innate ability to connect with people and help them to tell their stories. *Becoming Mum* is her first book.

First published in 2014 by
Liberties Press
140 Terenure Road North | Terenure | Dublin 6W
T: +353 (1) 405 5701| www.libertiespress.com | E: info@libertiespress.com

Trade enquiries to Gill & Macmillan Distribution
Hume Avenue | Park West | Dublin 12
T: +353 (1) 500 9534 | F: +353 (1) 500 9595 | E: sales@gillmacmillan.ie

Distributed in the United Kingdom by
Turnaround Publisher Services
Unit 3 | Olympia Trading Estate | Coburg Road | London N22 6TZ
T: +44 (0) 20 8829 3000 | E: orders@turnaround-uk.com

Distributed in the United States by
International Publishers Marketing
22841 Quicksilver Dr | Dulles, VA 20166
T: +1 (703) 661-1586 | F: +1 (703) 661-1547 | E: ipmmail@presswarehouse.com

ISBN: 978-1-909718-28-9
2 4 6 8 10 9 7 5 3 1

A CIP record for this title is available from the British Library.

Cover design by Liberties Press
Internal design by Liberties Press

Becoming Mum

How to Survive Childbirth and the Early Months of Motherhood

Kate Carbery

To Simon, Elizabeth and David

Contents

Acknowledgements

I have never been so affected by anything as I was by the birth of my first baby. Struggling to survive those early days, I reached out after two weeks through an online forum for new mothers. There was little support locally for women who didn't breastfeed, so we started our own group. I will be forever grateful to those women I met week in, week out, for the support and comfort they provided just by sharing that time with me. Many of them have contributed to the book. Having experienced the support of this new mothers' group, I had the idea to help other new mothers with this book. Several years later, many of us continue to support each other as close friends. Thank you Gemma McAnaney, Ita O'Sullivan, Aine Kane and Paula Durham for your continued friendship and encouragement to write *Becoming Mum*.

I interviewed over forty wonderful women and a few of their (just as wonderful) partners for this book. I am indebted to them all for answering some very personal questions and for their honesty in doing so. It's not always easy to admit it if parenthood doesn't deliver the warm and fuzzy experience we hoped for. Because of their input, this book will help to support new mothers as they embark on their journey.

When I had the idea to write *Becoming Mum*, I was overwhelmed by the encouragement I received from my family. I am lucky enough to have siblings who are among my closest friends. They never doubted that I could do this. Thank you Genevieve, Sarah, Emma, Jer and Mary Lys for your enthusiasm and positivity.

My parents never even blinked an eye when I told them that I wanted to write a book. Thanks Mum and Dad.

Through the arrivals of and early months with both of my children, I had enormous support from my friends and extended family who already had children or were having kids at the same time. They were part of the inspiration for this book. Their enthusiasm for *Becoming Mum* has been a great motivation on the days when it all seemed a bit hard. In particular, thank you to Aeidín McCarter, Roisín Moloney, Becca Carbery, Sheila Brennan, Liz McGauley, Rebecca Sheridan, Gavin O'Connor and Gwenda Jeffreys-Jones.

Keeping your sense of humour and perspective is so hard when you are submerged in new-baby-ville, and I am very lucky to have people to remind me of the pre-baby me. Thank you Jo Noble, Maria Donohoe and Deirdre Farrell for this. Please don't ever stop reminding me.

Thank you to Ita O'Sullivan for researching and providing much of the statistical information that is included in the book and for your unending enthusiasm and encouragement. John Butterly, your tough love and professional advice was gratefully received, thank you.

Thank you to Anne Atkinson, a night nurse and professional nanny, who, apart from helping me after the birth of my second baby, has contributed a few little gems of advice of her own.

A huge thank you to Seán O'Keeffe and the team at Liberties Press for their interest in my idea.

Thank you also to Olivia O'Leary for her honest and insightful foreword as well as her encouragement to write *Becoming Mum* in the first place. I am grateful to have a contribution from such an inspirational Irish woman and a warm, wonderful fellow mother.

Finally, to my own family: I feel very fortunate to have a husband who believes in me much more than I believe in myself.

Thank you Simon for helping me to make this happen. Elizabeth and David, you two have taught me so much. Thank you Elizabeth for your understanding as I ran out to do another interview just after bedtime. Forgive me for plonking you in front of the TV for an hour while I interviewed someone in the kitchen (although I know you enjoyed it). David, thank you for not arriving in this world before your due date, thus allowing me to finish the first draft. Thank you also for reminding me of the challenges of childbirth and those early months to include in this book. Somehow I had forgotten them.

Foreword

When I had my first and only baby, it was without any doubt the best and most exciting thing that had ever happened to me. Waking in the night, I'd hear a rustle in the cot beside me and feel dizzy with happiness. I was also fiercely protective. 'You and me against the world, kid,' I'd say, and sometimes it felt like that.

Because when you have your first baby, it seems like everyone in the world knows better than you do how care for it. At least, that's how they make you feel. When the wonderful midwives in the Coombe Hospital sent me home, with lots of encouragement, I felt reasonably secure. The months after that saw a slow erosion of confidence, partly because I was on my own most of the day with a small baby, and partly because the state's mother-and-baby services seemed to see themselves more as inspectors and critics of new mothers rather than as a support to them.

It still seems extraordinary to me that new mothers so often spend all day alone with a new small baby. This is the time when they most need physical and emotional support. Exhaustion and soreness from the birth itself is made worse by lack of sleep. Doctors will often say, as mine did repeatedly, 'Pregnancy is not a disease', as though that should in itself banish the discomfort of being pregnant and the pain, and sometimes the trauma, of child-birth. Very often new babies have colic or feeding complications and cry a great deal. Handling all that and trying to do basic housework add to one's sense of inadequacy. I believe strongly in paid paternity leave so that fathers can take over housekeeping duties for the first few months. If not, you need family or friends to step in, or you pay someone to help with the housework.

I will always remember answering the door to the visiting state-registered nurse when my baby was about two and a half months old. The baby had woken early and been fed and had gone back to sleep, and it was now mid-morning and I was still in my dressing gown. She first criticised me for not being properly up and dressed. Then she asked me if I was going back to work when my maternity leave was up. I said I was. She said that was a 'selfish' decision but if I was going to go back to work I should not put my child in a crèche or nursery. I replied with some asperity that that was a decision I would make myself but she continued to lecture me. By the time she left, she gave me the impression that she thought I was a slatternly, inadequate mother who was going back to work for 'selfish' reasons. So much for support and encouragement. Luckily she made me feel angry rather than depressed. I still feel angry now.

I wish I had known back then that I wasn't the only new mother who felt inadequate and misunderstood. I wish I had demanded the help and support I needed to cope at home. And I wish I had my visiting nurse back to be able to tell her that by undermining me, she was undermining the most important person in that small baby's life.

There has long been a conspiracy to make mothers feel that way, that because motherhood is the most natural thing in the world, it is effortless. Of course it isn't. Pregnancy and childbirth temporarily disrupt your body, and sometimes your mind. You have done something wonderful. You have produced another human being. How could it not take its toll?

What Kate Carbery has done in this book is to let new mothers themselves describe what it is like to have a baby. They highlight some of the difficulties would-be mothers should prepare for, and they provide reassurance for those who feel they should be handling it all better. They are frank and funny and unsentimental, and their advice is practical.

They present motherhood as it is: a great challenge, and an even greater joy.

Olivia O'Leary
March 2014

Olivia O'Leary has presented television and radio programmes over the years for both RTÉ and the BBC, including BBC's Newsnight *and RTÉ's* Prime Time. *She does a weekly political column for RTÉ Radio 1's* Drivetime. *Two collections of her radio columns have been published by The O'Brien Press.*

Introduction

Maybe you have always known you would become a mother. Maybe this decision to have a baby was a recent one. Maybe this is all a bit of a surprise. Whatever way you have come to motherhood, it is, without a doubt, one of the most intense, life-changing experiences you will ever go through. No matter how many conversations you have with friends who have had kids, nothing can prepare you for the changes ahead. Every woman is different, every birth is different, every baby is different. You will cope with childbirth and motherhood in your own way.

Think of this book as a virtual mother-and-baby group on paper, to keep you going until you have the energy to find a real one or to trawl through the internet forums. I was lucky enough to find a wonderful group of new mothers very early on. This book is intended to be a reassuring voice to remind you that you're OK, you're not insane and that other mothers-to-be, and new mothers, have felt the same way as you do now.

One of the best supports I had before and after my baby was born was the regular, sometimes daily, phone calls from one of my best friends. When I told her about how tough I was finding it, she reassured me that she had thought the same. It was normal. That's all I wanted to know: it was normal. I wanted to know that I wasn't mad, I wasn't a bad mother. My husband and I were regular human beings who were (just about) coping. That was what she told me and that's just what I needed to hear. Thank God for friends like that. Not everyone is so lucky.

This book is intended to support new mothers, in a society

where we don't always talk about how difficult childbirth and those first few months can be. I have mostly interviewed mothers in Ireland, and some Irish mothers overseas. I have also spoken to a few fathers, to get their point of view. It's not a book about how to have the perfect birth, how to get your child into a routine, or the daily trials of wet/dirty nappy levels or dealing with cracked nipples. It's about the mad stuff: the obsessive thoughts, the negative thoughts, alongside the joy and elation. It's about the fear of childbirth and the effects of sleep deprivation. It's not a fun book, but it's not heavy, and it's written in a way that makes it easy to read. Who has the energy to read lengthy books in those early months?

I was lucky enough to meet Anne Atkinson, who describes herself as a professional nanny, night nurse to newborns, sleep trainer to toddlers – who think night-time is the time to party – and a weaning and feeding advisor. She is often a shoulder to cry on, giving support and advice and encouragement to new parents. With over ten years' experience helping the parents of about a hundred babies and toddlers, she has kindly given her top tips at the end of some of the chapters.

The opinions and advice in this book are those of the interviewees. I've also described my own experience at the beginning of each chapter. *Becoming Mum* is not a substitute for professional medical advice. If you feel that you need professional help, I hope that the 'Resources and Useful Contacts' chapter at the end of the book will help you to find it. Many of the women and men interviewed opted for an alias, so that they could be completely honest in their answers. The ages of the parents given are the ages at the time of interview. Some of them have had their babies only recently, while others have children who are well into their teenage years. They are all real people with real experiences.

On a final note, every woman interviewed was asked whether their baby had been worth the often difficult transition to motherhood. Every single woman said yes.

The advice in this book is personal opinion taken from interviews and not the advice of the author. You should always seek medical advice from your GP, midwife or consultant if you are concerned about your or your baby's health.

1.
The Birth

Interviewees were asked about their hopes for childbirth and their actual experience of those births. Only five of the forty women I spoke to felt that the birth went as expected. Most of them had a very different experience to what they expected or hoped for. Those who had a detailed birth plan generally found that it didn't go to plan at all. As one mother put it, 'The baby writes the birth plan, not you.'

In this chapter, birth stories are listed under headings depending on whether the birth was with little or no pain relief, with an epidural, by caesarean section, by VBAC (vaginal birth after caesarean) or a home birth.

When I was having my first baby, one of the questions I kept asking people was, 'What does a contraction actually feel like?' It turns out that, as with most of these questions, it's different for everyone and can vary hugely from pregnancy to pregnancy depending on how the baby presents itself, and many other factors. I have listed their answers near the end of the chapter.

I also asked some fathers for their input about how they experienced the birth.

Births with Minimal Pain Relief

Kate, Age 38, Dublin

On the birth of my first baby, I was induced due to high blood pressure. I had hoped to have a drug-free labour. However, the induction was so intense I asked for an epidural. The anaesthetist was called but I was progressing too quickly and had to go ahead with gas and air. If I was being induced again, I'd definitely have an epidural. If I wasn't, I'd still try and go ahead with gas and air and see how it goes. The most painful part of the birth for me was the baby's head coming out (crowning). I really wish I'd done those awful perineal massage exercises they told us about; it would have helped that stretching a lot.

On my second, I felt much better prepared and went with the community midwife scheme at my local hospital, again planning a drug-free birth. My labour went brilliantly at first, still bloody sore, but it went smoothly until he got stuck in the birth canal, as he was presenting in a funny position and was 10 pounds 15 ounces. It ended up being an assisted birth: on my back, feet in stirrups, with an episiotomy and ventouse delivery. It wasn't what I had hoped for, but I knew this time around to expect anything, that the baby would dictate the birth.

A lot of people these days are anti-hospitals when it comes to childbirth. I believe that a midwife-led birth within a hospital is ideal. If it wasn't for those doctors who arrived at the end and helped deliver my baby, God knows what would have happened. Even two very experienced, talented midwives couldn't get us there.

Caroline, Age 35, Dublin

Caroline had a birth plan on her first baby. She had hoped to deliver naturally but as she went ten days over, she was advised to come in to hospital to be induced. 'Being my first baby, I didn't realise that I had a choice, that I could have said no.' Labour kicked in very quickly and it was very intense. Her midwife was very encouraging and supportive of her birth plan but told her it could be hours, or a lot longer, before the baby arrived. All of a sudden, they said the baby was in distress, that they needed to get him out. They told her to lie back, and the stirrups shot up.

'It was just what I didn't want, I was kicking my legs out of them . . . I was screaming my head off and the doctor was telling me to stop screaming and push.' They said they needed to do an episiotomy, which she also didn't want, but then the baby was born using a ventouse. The midwife asked her afterwards if she wanted to talk about what had happened. 'I was so angry with her. That birth was not what I wanted and she just flipped me over and put my legs in these things . . . it felt so unnatural to give birth on my back.' If she was doing it again she would have insisted on not being induced at ten days if the scan showed that the baby was still doing OK.

Her second birth was completely different. She had no birth plan and he was also ten days over. The doctor recommended her to be induced and she said no, as she had just been told there was lots of fluid and the scan was fine. The doctor said, 'Well, if it was my baby I wouldn't be putting my own wishes for some sort of birth that I want over the safety of the baby.' She went naturally at twelve days overdue and had the kind of birth she had hoped for with her first with no interventions.

Elaine, Age 29, Dublin

Elaine's daughter was born in hospital in Dublin, and the experience was overall a positive one. She was happy to have had a drug-free labour, apart from some gas and air. Looking back, she realised that she didn't have enough knowledge and practice of how to breathe during labour. She believes that doing the breathing correctly would have helped a lot. It wasn't as scary as she thought it would be, and she had forgotten about the pain by the next day.

Sara, Age 39, Dublin

Sara was delighted to be on the community midwife scheme at her local hospital, hoping for a natural labour and a short hospital visit. When they did eventually get to hospital after a long labour at home, the midwife-led suite was full, as was the backup ward due to it being an incredibly busy night. 'I basically got shoved into a toilet in the back of the hospital!' None of the community midwives were available, so one of the regular midwives took charge and kept suggesting an epidural despite the labour progressing well. She had to fight for her plan to have a natural birth. Thankfully the community midwives ended up being present at the birth, and they were brilliant. 'They got me through it . . . I really had to stop that other midwife pushing the epidural. It was obvious she didn't want to deal with a woman who wasn't medicated during labour . . . A good midwife is absolutely fundamental.' She feels that part of the problem was that this new midwife saw her at her weakest and most tired moment, whereas the community midwives knew her and knew what she was capable of. She believes that it's at this weak point that you need these midwives who know what you are like and can get you past that point where you feel you just can't go on. 'I felt very satisfied that I did it, and I did it the way I wanted to, and she's here and she's safe. I just wanted to go home then.'

Laoise, Age 37, Dublin

Laoise planned a home birth for both of her children. On her first, she had laboured well at home but because there was meconium in her waters she had to be brought to the hospital as a precautionary measure in the back of the car on all fours at ten centimetres dilated. She had the baby thirty minutes after arriving in the hospital. 'It wasn't a negative experience going to the hospital.' Her reasons for home birth were more about the after-care of a home birth than birthing at home. 'When I was pregnant, I really wanted to know what childbirth was like, so I read everything. I had a lot of contact hours with my midwife and she would be with me for two hours chatting. I didn't know why she was always here so long, but she was actually giving me the confidence and knowledge to be able to do it . . . I was always keenly listening if people would say that labour was OK, but never once did anyone suggest that it wasn't hard. It is hard, but it's doable.'

People used to try to make her feel better about the fact that she had to go to the hospital as if they thought she had failed. 'I wasn't really disappointed. It was the safest way to have the baby and I got to labour at home. I got one-to-one care from someone who knew me and knew my disposition.'

Astrid, Age 39, Germany/Dublin

Astrid's first baby was born in Germany, and her second in Dublin. She had no birth plan and no major expectations about the birth of her first daughter. She was induced because the labour didn't start properly.

Her husband was in Ireland and catching the next plane, and due to arrive there at 6 PM. 'They wanted to induce me at 3 o'clock in the afternoon. I wasn't strong enough to say no . . . .They really frightened me in the hospital.' They went ahead with the induction at 3 PM. Interestingly, the labour kicked in, with very intense contractions, as soon as her husband arrived. 'I had to push for an hour. There were a few complications. My daughter was very big, her shoulder got stuck so they thought they might have to do a caesarean section. It was a very stressful labour . . . and a very traumatic birth for my daughter and for my husband.' Finally the shoulder was released and she was born. 'I was shocked by it. There were three midwives sitting on me pushing her out, doing a leg manoeuvre trying to get the shoulder out. My husband thought it was very medieval.' She remembers that the shock lasted about a week.

She knew that she wanted to give birth differently the second time, if possible. She wanted to try different positions, and had her second daughter while kneeling. It all went as hoped and she was so much happier after it despite still being exhausted. She had no pain relief as her daughter was born very quickly, having laboured well at home. She noticed how happy she was in the weeks afterwards, as it had all gone so well. If she were to go back to her first birth, she would follow her own instinct more. If it was safe for the baby, she would have fought the decision on the induction with more confidence.

Sarah, Age 37, Cork/London

Sarah didn't have a specific birth plan on her first baby; she tried not to speculate about how the birth would be. 'I tried not to think too much about the birth. I was never too worried about the pain, you just have to get on with it . . . I had always thought it would be nice to do without pain relief.' Her first baby was ten days early, which she didn't expect. She was fully dilated when she arrived at the hospital, and that was a bit of a shock. 'The pain was pretty full-on but when I was told I was fully dilated there was quite a lot of relief . . . but still you're shocked at how much it does hurt, how it comes in waves and how much you need to control it.' On subsequent births she was surprised by how painful the contractions were even only at two centimetres dilated. She now knows she progresses very quickly, so the contractions were quite intense.

She found the pushing part the hardest. 'Even on my third baby, you would think the pushing would be easier, but that was the most difficult one for me, maybe because he was bigger.' She found that after the head came out, it was hard to push further to get the rest of the baby out and then find the energy to push the placenta out.

Rachel, Age 41, Dublin

Rachel never thought she could have children, and was thrilled to be pregnant. She had no birth plan, as she felt there was no point in having one because you just don't know what is going to happen. The doctor was eager to get the baby out, as she had developed some complications with her liver. They scheduled her for induction at thirty-nine weeks. While she waited for the induction to start, she was getting some cramps. 'I cramped the whole way through my pregnancy so I didn't remark on any of the cramps I was feeling', which were a bit stronger than usual. She told the doctor about the cramping and when they checked her, her cervix was already softening naturally. They tried to break her waters and there was just a dribble instead of the big splash she'd expected. 'I wanted the Hollywood version and I didn't get it!' She was told she wouldn't give birth till the next afternoon at the earliest. After her contractions kicked in, they checked her again and 'they told me I was *nearly* what they consider being in labour, which is about two centimetres.' An hour later the head sister came in and asked her to keep it down a bit. 'Then my waters broke and then I got Hollywood! I went straight from two centimetres to fully dilated in that hour.' They ran to the delivery ward with her in a wheelchair. 'We got to the delivery ward at 3.14 PM and the baby was born at 3.20 PM . . . it was the most intense experience of my entire life.'

Yvonne, Age 40, Dublin

Yvonne was twenty-one having her first baby, and she found it terrifying. Her mother was with her: 'If I hadn't had her, I think I would have lost it.' She was really embarrassed. 'There were about four male doctors down below looking at me . . . You're not told any of this.' She was shocked at the fact that you can have a bowel movement during labour. 'It's a natural thing that can happen – that's what I would have liked to have known.'

She was thirty-one having her second baby, and it was like being a new mother all over again. Her husband was with her for the births of her second and third babies. When they realised she needed to go to the hospital, 'he went and had a quick shave and on the third one he said he wanted to have a quick shower. Men just don't have a clue!'

Tracey, Age 38, Roscommon

Tracey had a clear plan in her head when she was having her first baby. She had learned a lot about the medicalisation of childbirth during her nursing studies and felt she wanted as little medical intervention as possible. 'I was induced at 6 AM . . . and the nurse said it usually takes a few days . . . Within forty minutes I started in to ferocious contractions . . . It pretty much went to three minutes apart after two hours of starting the induction process.' She had anticipated a slower lead-in to the pain rather than the immediate intensity of the contractions. 'They are definitely more intense with the induction . . . It just felt all wrong . . . Your own hormones are supposed to kick in, your own natural pain relief is supposed to kick in . . . but it all felt fake . . . I should have taken the epidural at that point . . . Then they hooked me up to the tracer and I felt like a caged animal . . . I needed to pace and I couldn't pace.'

Finally she asked for the epidural but she didn't feel that she could stay still long enough for it to be safely administered. As she wasn't progressing, they administered oxytocin and she rocketed from six centimetres to ten centimetres in an hour and then started to push. She pushed for an hour with six people in the room, which she found unsettling. 'Then I got really distressed with pooing. I just didn't really realise that I would poo, I was so naive about so many things . . . it felt like it was coming forever, and it was stinking!' She felt she was probably holding back because she was trying to stop pooing, which made it more painful. She didn't connect with the young midwife and felt she needed more direction from someone more experienced who knew her better.

She wishes that she had been less rigid in her birth plan and asked for the epidural earlier than she did, as the induction was so intense. She approached her subsequent birth very differently. 'I had no birth plan, we would just take whatever came . . . In the end I did have a natural birth with my second baby, and yeah, it hurts, there's no two ways about it, but I wasn't scared . . . I was terrified the whole way through the first time.' Second time round, Tracey also had a midwife who knew her, and her birth history, as well as a doula. It was a much more positive experience. 'A lot of it is how you cope with it. If you can get rid of the fear factor . . . The fear suppresses the natural pain relief.'

Kathleen, Age 38, Donegal

Kathleen had no birth plan for either of her babies' births. She hadn't expected her labour to go on so long: in total, it was about forty-eight hours. The only request she did have was that she didn't want pethidine as it makes her very nauseous. Despite having been clear about this, 'I still had to tell them several times. Luckily my husband was well aware that I didn't want it.'

'What I found difficult was the fact that there seemed to be no end in sight to the pain . . . At one point I asked the midwife how long this was going to go on, and she didn't answer me. I told her it was quite all right for her to tell me a lie, but I needed some sort of goal to get to.' She found that having a goal to work towards helped her get through the pain of labour.

Fionnuala, Age 40, Dublin

Fionnuala felt that a hypno-birthing course she did helped her a lot during labour, helping her to face the fear of childbirth. She wanted to find a way to feel more empowered approaching labour. She read once that if a woman isn't a goddess giving birth, someone's not supporting her. 'I really believe that. If you think about it, women were worshipped for it . . . It's so amazing.' She had a birth plan, in order to help her feel in control. When she told her consultant that she had done hypno-birthing, he said, 'Oh, these hypno-birthers have very long labours.' She felt confident that it would go well and didn't bother arguing with him. 'It went fine. I had all this body preparation, constantly imagining that it was going to be really easy, not painful and fast. And it was.' She believes that if you are afraid, your body responds to that fear. On her way to hospital once contractions had started, she remembered a tip from a friend and started thinking 'I can get through this minute . . . It's all about being in the moment.'

When discussing her birth plan with her consultant, they discussed her wish not to have an episiotomy as she knew that there were ways that the medical team could help prevent one. 'He said, what do you think we do, cut people open for the fun?' Her approach to childbirth was to curl up and try to block out the lights and activity in the hospital and focus on her guided meditation. 'Things started moving really quickly . . . I vomited a lot . . . I started doing my yoga exercises . . . I didn't want my husband anywhere near me.' Her contractions were coming every thirty seconds. They didn't believe her, and when the midwife finally checked her, they found that she had almost fully dilated in three hours, and brought her straight to the delivery room. 'One thing that makes me want to have a home birth is that shift from the ante-natal room to the delivery room . . . It just took me out of it again; I just wasn't comfortable.'

She knows she was on the path of feeling really empowered and confident, but that last part made her lose the self-belief that she could do it. She had an episiotomy in the end, and that caused her a lot of pain afterwards, as it was quite long.

Anna, Age 37, Dublin

Anna attended a private ante-natal course rather than the hospital one, and felt she got much broader advice about the birth than the hospital one. Having spoken to friends, she knew that all births are completely different. She decided to have a loose birth plan with two things on it that she didn't want: pethidine and an epidural. 'I had to lie to the nurse to not get pethidine. I told them I was intolerant to it. If I hadn't said that I would have had to argue with her.' She felt that anything she wanted to do outside of the hospital's norm was fought against, whether that be giving birth in any position other than on her back or taking pethidine. 'The other thing that nobody ever mentions is that you can end up peeing, pooing and vomiting during labour. I only knew because my friend had told me.'

Heather, Age 39, Dublin

Heather and her partner felt that it was unwise to have a set birth plan. However, there were two things that she knew she didn't want: to give birth on her back, and an episiotomy. In the end she had both. Her labour progressed quite quickly, as she was in a dark ward during the night, and she felt this helped a lot. When she got to the delivery room, there were very bright lights and a medical student she had never met. She felt that this didn't help with the progression of labour. She wasn't offered any position other than lying on her back. 'On the third push, the baby was crowning. It should have been one more push but then it stopped for an hour and twenty minutes . . . I think my body just said no it's not safe to give birth here with the bright lights, and strangers in the room.' She was very relieved after the birth that he had arrived safely, and was very grateful to the midwives. 'I've never felt traumatised by it. It's only now in the cold light of day, looking back . . . I think that should have gone differently.'

Heather used a relaxation CD with techniques to visualise getting through the contractions. 'I really used them at the time; it's the only thing that stopped me panicking. At one point I had a feeling of panic because the contractions were getting so strong and I thought "I can't do this" . . . it clicked into place . . . it definitely kept me very calm.'

In retrospect, she would have liked it if she had had the environment that had been promised to her before the birth, i.e. giving birth in a different position, dim lighting, and a birthing ball. She would have prefered it if her husband had not had to be the other prop for her legs. 'I think it was very distressing for him and of course he saw more than I did.' She would also now consider a home birth after her hospital experience.

Marie, Age 49, Dublin

Marie had her first child in hospital, but her second birth was a home birth. The hospital birth was not a positive experience. She had absolutely expected a natural birth and had written a birth plan. She was adamant about all the things she didn't want to happen. She knows now that she needed to labour at home for longer but she feels in retrospect that the hospital needed her to fit in with their schedule, which is why they broke her waters. When they did break her waters, 'not only was it physically unpleasant, I remember feeling, this isn't right actually.' It also didn't help her labour to progress any faster. They administered oxytocin to help it along. 'My next memory is lying on the table and them saying, 'She's in distress, you have to hurry up', and me saying, 'I can't hurry up!' I was coping pretty well with the pain but as 5 PM approached they suggested an epidural even though she was progressing gradually – but too slowly, she feels, for the hospital staff.

They ended up performing an episiotomy without asking her, and using a ventouse to deliver the baby. 'The consultant was so unpleasant, he obviously was to clock out at five and I was holding him up.'

Helena, Age 33, Dublin

Unlike her first birth, Helena wasn't induced on the birth of her second baby. As a result, the pains were more manageable, with longer gaps in between. She didn't have a birth plan and was open to whatever happened. She ended up having a natural birth (despite wanting an epidural, she couldn't get one in the end!) and it went fine. She was glad in the end that she had done it with no pain relief.

Births with Epidurals

Kerry, Age 37, Dublin

Kerry had expected a natural childbirth with no pain relief. She was awake all night in early labour and was exhausted when she finally asked for it. 'The epidural was the best thing. I'm such a convert, I had thought I would be paralysed or something.' She didn't regret asking for it. She felt she really needed it, and would have it again if she had another baby.

Helena, Age 33, Dublin

Like many new mothers, Helena had a birth plan for her first baby which included a natural birth with little or no pain relief. 'I was very frustrated when things didn't go as I wanted.' Due to low levels of fluid around the baby, she was induced, and couldn't cope with only gas and air, as the contractions were so intense. It went on for quite a long time. She wanted to avoid the epidural, as she was worried about something going wrong and being paralysed. However, she became so exhausted she decided to go for it, as she needed to sleep and knew she couldn't keep going without it. 'It was the right thing to do. I could relax and take a few naps.'

Cathy, Age 30, Dublin

From early on, the birth of Cathy's first baby was a little complicated. She was put on her back and told not to move off her back. 'It was just a run of bad events. I came in and there was loads of meconium in the waters, so they wanted to monitor it. They couldn't keep track of her heartbeat, so they wanted me to stay really, really still so that they could.' It was a long labour: she was not progressing beyond a couple of centimetres dilated for six or seven hours, and her baby was facing the wrong way around. The contractions were very intense and strong. Once she was told she couldn't move at all, due to the need to monitor her, she went for the epidural. She felt she was in the best place being in the hospital and was happy to put her trust in the medical team. Oxytocin was administered, as she wasn't progressing, but the epidural worked really well and she didn't feel anything up to eight centimetres dilation. Then the epidural wore off and the pains of the contractions became more real. 'I just remember repeating, "They're going to give me another epidural, right?"' She tried to push, to no avail. They tried forceps but they didn't work. They gave her some pethidine and gave her another hour, asked her to push and tried the ventouse. The ventouse amazed her, the doctor had his foot up on the bed as he tried to 'suck' the baby out, and then her baby was born. She didn't mind the interventions in the birth and had always known it wouldn't be a walk in the park.

Ella, Age 45, Dublin

Ella didn't have a birth plan on any of her births; she just wanted to go with whatever the consultant felt was the best. 'He asked me about the birth plan and I said really just get the babies out alive. He said, "That's the best plan I've ever come across."' Her first boy was a vaginal delivery and her twins were born by caesarean. She had been told that your waters don't normally break early like you see on TV, which only happens in about 10 percent of cases. However, it happened to her at thirty-seven weeks on a train platform. She had waited a long time for her first baby, so despite feeling embarrassed, she was excited. She didn't want to take the epidural too early and held out till near the end of a long labour and fell asleep once it kicked in. 'I couldn't get the baby out. The consultant was popping in and out of the room, very respectful of the midwives' role, but then he decided that the baby had to come out.' They gave an episiotomy and used a ventouse to get the baby out. She was fine with how the birth went and was happy to trust the consultant's decisions.

Mary, Age 32, Tipperary

Mary read every book that she could find, and was no clearer when the time came about whether she was going into labour or not. 'I thought I was going into labour every night from about six weeks before; with every twinge I thought I had started.' She was very positive about the birth, had done yoga and practised her breathing techniques. 'I didn't watch any birthing programmes . . . I didn't want to know all the gory details, and what could go wrong. I thought I would just go in and hope for the best . . . I was open to the epidural and pain relief, whatever got me through.' She had initially thought she would go naturally, but six weeks before the birth she was in hospital for a couple of nights and, having listened to women in labour, she decided to be more open to the idea of an epidural. When she finally did go into labour, she ended up having her waters broken and oxytocin administered, as she wasn't dilating. The severity of the contractions led to her accepting the epidural. Her yoga breathing made a huge difference and helped her through the contractions and to feel more in control. The epidural definitely took away a lot of the pain, and she felt 'quite comfortable' when she was pushing. It meant she could have a rest after many hours of very painful contractions. She had an episiotomy also, and was very nervous about it but didn't feel a thing. She was on a high once the baby arrived and was so happy that the pregnancy was over and the baby was there safely. 'The day after I had her, someone asked me if I would do it all again, and I couldn't answer them, but now I know that I would.'

Ruth, Age 36, Kildare

On her first baby, Ruth said she was 'deluded' with her ideas of what childbirth would be like. She was only nineteen having her first baby and was quite unprepared. She hadn't read anything and hadn't spoken to many people about childbirth. 'I should have prepared more. I didn't do my homework, I was young and naive.' What she remembers hating the most was the lack of control. She opted for an epidural, which meant she felt even less in control. Her experience on the next two babies was totally different. She had done more research, had planned what she wanted, and gave birth to one of them standing up. In both cases she had no pain relief. They used aromatherapy oils and her husband helped relieve the pain through acupuncture pressure points.

Megan, Age 40, Dublin

Megan had no birth plan, and found the birth to be easier than expected. The pain that she felt during contractions was like a stronger version of the pain she felt the day before her period. She took an epidural a lot quicker than expected when the pain really kicked in. 'The pushing was hard, I was pushing for an hour and I felt like my eyes were coming out, and I was fearful of being ripped.' She only had two stitches, and no episiotomy, despite having a 9 pound 14 ounce baby. She was very happy with how the birth went.

Deirdre, Age 40, Dublin

Deirdre didn't have a birth plan for either of her babies' births. She didn't particularly want an epidural but was open to it if she needed it. Her first birth was very quick, but went fine. On her second baby, her blood pressure went up and they started talking about inducing her. She started worrying, as it was so different from her first birth and they weren't talking to her about it. 'The communication was appalling; they just don't treat you like you're human. You're an adult, a well-educated woman who just needed the information and then could probably deal with the situation a lot better.' After multiple applications of gel to induce labour, she was tired and just wasn't in the right place mentally to go ahead with a labour without an epidural.

Isobel, Age 39, Dublin

Isobel has a low pain threshold and had planned on an epidural but it didn't work on her first baby. All the pain was in her back, and she found it unbearable. The nurses gave her pethidine without asking her. 'I've never done drugs but I'd imagine it's like you're buzzing on about five ecstasy tablets over in Ibiza; it makes you go into another world.' The epidural worked on her second and she felt nothing. 'It's like getting your toes painted.'

Although she was really worried about the pain of childbirth, and used to always worry about dying in childbirth, she remembers being more concerned about how she looked during childbirth. 'Will I look nice in the bed? Will my husband love me when I'm pushing the baby out?' She remembers shouting at her husband during the birth to stop wiping her face with a facecloth, because he was wiping her makeup off. 'If I'd only known that I'd probably never wear makeup again for the next four years!' Worrying about the pain had been a secondary concern beforehand, as she assumed the epidural would do its thing. 'I had this image of the birth and motherhood as a page out of a baby catalogue. I never worried about vomit, blood, mucous, poo, pain, sleeplessness.'

Caesarean Births

Rebecca, Age 41, Kilkenny

When Rebecca was having her first baby, she thought she had a pretty good idea of how it would go; waters would break during the night, she wouldn't be induced, she would have no pain relief and no intervention from doctors. Instead, she had a caesarean, because her baby's head hadn't engaged and she was two weeks overdue. Her second baby was also a section, despite her doctor saying there was no reason she shouldn't have a vaginal delivery. She experienced intense labour pains for about five hours but didn't dilate. 'I was crying once the epidural kicked in . . . it was such a relief.'

Emma, Age 44, Athy

Emma described the caesarean as though 'you're sitting in the car and someone is changing the wheel. You can feel the pulling and the tugging but you can't physically feel it. Then they hand you the baby.'

Barbara, Age 32, Dublin

Barbara's now two-year-old twin boys were born in hospital in

Dublin after an emergency caesarean due to the presenting twin being in footling breech position (feet/foot first). Although people might have expected her to be in shock, as she had planned a vaginal delivery, she actually felt OK about it. The decision had been taken out of her hands.

What is a caesarean really like? 'It's the same as everybody says: you have no idea what's happening down there, you can't see anything, all you can feel is rummaging . . . It's not unpleasant.' The speed at which the babies were taken out once the surgery began really surprised her – it only took a matter of minutes.

Barbara feels that a danger of the early days is that you have made up your mind about how birth and the days that follow will be. However, it's not really possible to know what will happen until the time comes.

Sinead, Age 37, Cork

On her first baby, Sinead waited until she was twenty days overdue and then felt she had no choice but to accept her consultant's recommendation that she be induced. 'I wasn't particularly happy about it, but I was resigned to it. He was a big baby, but nobody had explained to me that having such a big baby might be a problem.' They put her on oxytocin to induce labour. 'I hadn't realised that being on a drip was going to be so intense . . . I had wanted a natural birth and didn't want any painkillers.' She feels that if you're going to be induced, it should go hand in hand with pain relief because it's not a natural birth. Her husband had learned lots of acupressure techniques and she did a lot of yoga breathing and felt that was sufficient for quite a while. 'After seven hours on the drip, I was very tired, physically and mentally wrecked. It wasn't till I got to seven hours that I felt that the pain was too much.' She stayed at two centimetres for all that time. Things were not progressing. She opted for an epidural, as she realised that even if labour did progress, she'd never have the energy to go without pain relief. She was terrified of a needle in her spine, but it was OK. They didn't want her husband in the room when the needle was going in; she doesn't know why. He had been a very active birth partner up to that point, so she found his absence difficult.

The baby's heart rate dropped every time she had a contraction, and the consultant told her he wanted to do a caesarean. 'So I went all the way from thinking I would have a yogic natural birth to having probably the most intervention you could possibly have.' In hindsight, she thinks that it would be useful to explain to pregnant women that 'if you have to be induced, and things don't progress, and you have a large baby and there are all these indicators, you need to have it in your mind that you might end up with a caesarean section.'

She cried on her way to the operating theatre, as she was disappointed with how it had gone, but knew it was what needed to happen at that stage. They put a curtain up, but did offer for her to see it on a screen – which she declined! They had to shave some of her pubic hair, as the cut was being made very close to her pubic area. The sensation was one of rummaging and tugging but it was not painful. She felt like the baby was 'a very separate thing to me' in comparison to her next delivery, which was natural and where the baby felt like it was a part of her. 'It was a sort of out-of-body, separate experience. It felt like my head was in one place and my body in another.' Looking back now, she has a lot more perspective on it. 'I now think how lucky we both are to be here . . . OK it wasn't an ideal way to give birth, but I feel lucky. It's hard to have perspective on it in the first few weeks and months after it.'

Deborah, Age 37, Dublin

Deborah's daughter was born in hospital in Dublin after an unexpected caesarean. 'It wasn't the birth I'd planned. It was a caesarean in the end . . . and I was induced. I'd hoped to avoid both those things.' She didn't dilate despite a lengthy induction process. 'I was a bit disappointed with how it went . . . I felt I was rushed.' She felt that maybe her body would have managed it if she had been given more time, as her waters had broken naturally. Hospital policy meant that she had to have the baby within twelve hours of the labour having started. She didn't feel traumatised by the process of undergoing a caesarean at the time, as her daughter arrived safely and that was the most important thing. However, looking back, she is disappointed that she didn't get to hold her daughter at all till 11 AM the next morning. This was due to the amount of medication she had taken for the birth and the restrictions of the old hospital building for access to the ICU by trolley or wheelchair.

A caesarean can bring with it various challenges, like the effects of the anaesthetic and having a catheter. 'You hear all these different things about birth, but it can rapidly shift up to being really medicalised.' She had lots of ideas before the birth about skin-to-skin contact and feeding her daughter herself. 'It wasn't perfect but who has the perfect birth?'

Alison, Age 38, Kildare/San Francisco

Alison's first baby was born by planned caesarean as she suffers from Crohn's disease. 'It was much more clinical than I thought it was going to be: there were two doctors, a bunch of nurses, a paediatrician and the anaesthesiologist.' The pain after the caesarean was pretty bad in the first few days. She describes it as a tight, burning feeling. She can't take a lot of heavy painkillers and was on just regular over-the-counter painkillers, so felt more pain than she maybe had to. 'Everything healed fine. There was minimum scarring, and the scar was very small.' The pain after her second caesarean was a lot less; she's not sure why. She was out of pain two days after the birth.

Michelle, Age 30, Dublin

Michelle was two weeks overdue but after a cervical sweep (manual stimulation of the cervix to release hormones which trigger labour) in hospital her contractions started very quickly. She had a birth plan which included not wanting pethidine, as she was worried the baby would be dopey or sleepy after it was born. However, due to the fact that she wasn't dilating yet, pethidine was all they offered her in terms of pain relief, and they assured her that she wasn't going to give birth for several hours, so the pethidine would have worn off. 'I thought about the reasons why I wouldn't take it, which were basically because my mum said I had to have a natural birth, and I thought, screw that. I took the pethidine and it was brilliant . . . I slept through my contractions and it started wearing off just as I was being brought to the labour ward.' She never dilated more than one centimetre despite oxytocin being administered. 'I was starting to get tired, so I took the epidural . . . Everything worked really well and I snoozed! It was actually a lovely experience!' They then advised that she have a caesarean section, as there was little or no fluid left around her baby and she wasn't progressing. 'They throw paperwork at you when you're in that state and you have to sign it . . . I couldn't believe the number of people in the theatre – about nine people altogether. It all happened so quickly.' She felt what helped her most to get through the contractions, apart from the pain relief administered, was the breathing she had practised.

Suzy, Age 36, Dublin

Suzy didn't have a birth plan, except that she was happy to 'bring on the drugs'. She had read everything she could find about giving birth. 'I knew from a medical perspective, go with whatever needs to be done at the time . . . I absolutely knew that whatever drugs were needed, get them into me . . . I want them and I want them twenty minutes ago.' She had two major concerns as she went into labour. Firstly, she was really worried that her bladder would not survive pregnancy, as she always needed to go to the loo regularly even before pregnancy. Secondly, she worried that her sexual capability would be damaged during childbirth and that sex with her husband just wouldn't be the same again. For this reason, she really hoped for a caesarean section.

As she was two weeks overdue, she was induced. The drugs kicked in very quickly. 'I knew induction was tough, but I didn't know how hard it was going to be . . . The contractions were coming hard and fast with no break . . . I roared the place down.' She remembers that the fear overcame the pain, that her whole body was consumed by the potential of the pain of the contraction coming back again. She got the epidural and once it took effect, she introduced herself to everyone in the room that she had been shouting at, and apologised profusely. It took four hours from then. She had a nap during that time, was woken by the midwife, and after four pushes the baby was born. She will never forget the pain before the epidural. 'It frightened me because there is that horrible feeling in you that you're not in control, your body is doing whatever it wants, and I'm just here for the journey . . . I was so scared of how big that was.'

Emma, Age 33, Dublin

Emma thinks she would have found it hard to get through her labour without her hypno-birthing CD; it was really helpful. She had a birth plan on her first baby, including not having her waters broken, no oxytocin and no epidural. However, she ended up having three days of contractions, not dilating fully and having a caesarean section. She had taken aspirin for back pain a few days before her labour started, but unfortunately this meant she couldn't have the epidural even a few days later.

On her second baby, she was planning on a vaginal delivery. She was twelve days over and despite the cervix softening and her starting to get pains, she wasn't dilating. Both first and second babies were facing the wrong way. 'I just know that the reason why me and my kids are here now, is because of caesarean sections.' She doesn't know how her babies could have been born otherwise. She partly felt that she hadn't given birth 'properly' as she hadn't had a vaginal delivery. 'I wanted to experience what everybody else experienced . . . Everyone else had gone in and pushed their babies out, what's wrong with me? I actually felt that it was my own fault that I ended up with a section, it was completely irrational.'

She found it hard after the caesarean section as she couldn't get out of bed, and couldn't get her babies out of the cot when they were crying. 'I remember the second night, I was a bit of an emotional wreck. I wrapped my son up in the blanket . . . It was wet. I couldn't understand how it could have been wet . . . Then I realised the pee had come out of his nappy. I was so deluded . . . I was exhausted, hallucinating in the night . . . You don't know where you are.'

Patricia, Age 35, Dublin

The birth of Patricia's first baby was very tough: a caesarean section after five nights of no sleep. 'I was all geared up for the natural birth, had done the yoga, done the hypnosis, bouncing on the yoga ball continuously . . . I started on a Saturday night and I eventually had my son on the Thursday by caesarean.' Her birth plan was all geared towards a natural birth. It included not having her waters broken, no epidural unless she requested it at least twice, and no oxytocin. After the birth, 'I definitely think I was in shock for quite a while afterwards. While I had an expectation that it would be tough, and even though when I was going through it I was calm and controlled, it was only afterwards that I actually felt that I had been hit by a train. Then at the end of all that I had an operation and was handed a baby that I didn't know what to do with and they said helpful things like "Trust your instincts!"'

'For a long time I was convinced to my core that there was no way I could possibly go through that again. It wasn't the pregnancy, or the baby, it was having the baby . . . It was horrendous.' Patricia had no frame of reference; she didn't know many people who had children. Even though she believes it's nice to go to the pregnancy yoga and be told you can manage it, 'You have to be open-minded and you have to anticipate that maybe it won't go the way that you expect it to go . . . As my consultant said, the baby writes the birth plan, not you.'

Julianne, Age 39, Tipperary

On her first baby, Julianne had a partial rupture of the membranes. This means that her waters broke partially, but the baby's head sealed it off again. As a result, the doctors were not prepared to leave her for more than twenty-four hours before inducing her. The induction caused a five-minute-long Braxton Hicks contraction and a resulting lower heart rate in her baby. That evening the doctors decided to take her to theatre for a caesarean. Julianne didn't mind, as she had discussed it previously with her consultant. She was, in fact, relieved.

Andrea, Age 38, Dublin

Andrea had no birth plan. Her first baby was breech so she knew she would be having a caesarean. 'It was all very surreal, very planned, like we were going on holidays.' However, the communication around what was happening and when it was going to happen was poor. When she was being taken away to be prepped for surgery, she thought it was an ante-chamber to the operating theatre. 'It turned out that it was actually the operating theatre.' Her husband was told to stay away until she was ready. She had to ask for him once she realised they were ready to start the procedure. She didn't find the procedure pleasant. 'I know lots of people opt for a c-section, and it's the easy approach, ' too posh to push ' and all that . . . Part of me was very relieved to have a c-section; I was really terrified about natural birth . . . but given the choice (her second child was a vaginal birth) there's no way I would elect to have surgery if I didn't have to. It's pretty major.' The medical staff seemed to be having a lot of difficulty getting the baby out, and they were getting anxious. Then she heard the consultant shouting 'This baby needs oxygen!' and the medical staff took the baby away without any reassurance for Andrea or her husband. She trusted the medical team and didn't doubt them, but it wasn't exactly pleasant. Her husband found it to be one of the most difficult experiences of his life.

She hadn't realised that she would be wheeled away to a recovery room and her husband 'was dumped in this little room, the nappy-changing area, with the baby in this wheelie cot, and the baby was crying because she wanted to be fed.'

Gemma, Age 40, Dublin

Gemma was eleven days overdue on her first baby and was booked in to be induced. After they broke her waters, her progress was very slow and both she and the baby developed a temperature; as a result, the baby had to be delivered by caesarean. 'I was quite happy, because actually you could hear screaming – soundproofing isn't part of the deal!' Her birth plan was to be open-minded.

On the public ward, the midwives were extremely busy and couldn't give her the support she needed. She got great care in the delivery suite and the High Dependency Unit, where she was for a day. She had lost a lot of blood. As soon as she got back to the public ward, she felt unsupported. In fact, she was told she was an 'anxious mum' by a midwife, when actually she feels that she was just a new mum, who didn't know what she was doing and needed help.

VBACs (Vaginal Births after Caesareans)

Sinead, Age 37, Cork

For her second delivery, Sinead was very hopeful that she could have a VBAC, having had a very difficult caesarean birth with her first baby. 'I didn't have any kind of presumption about it, but I felt really confident that it could happen . . . I wasn't going to be devastated and upset if it didn't.' Her consultant was quite firm about not letting her go overdue the second time around. On her first delivery she hadn't responded to being induced, the baby had been very big and a caesarean had been necessary in the end. At thirty eight weeks she went to an acupuncturist who specialised in inducing labour on overdue babies. She felt great after her acupuncture session, and five days before her due date she woke up and her contractions had started. 'I felt grateful to be having contractions, so the pain wasn't really a problem, I think pain is all in your attitude to it.' During labour she used her yoga breathing and postures. She felt she really did it her own way, and after five pushes the baby was out. She was so happy to have the kind of birth she hoped for and felt that she wasn't delivering the baby, her body was.

Gemma, Age 40, Dublin

For Gemma, having her second baby was a much calmer experience than her first, which was a caesarean birth. At the eighmonth mark, on her second, she banged her stomach just above the belly-button. It was very painful for a moment, but then she felt OK. 'I should have gone to the hospital, but I felt stupid, that it was only a tap. On my first pregnancy I went back and forth to the hospital a lot.' The bang kicked off labour but it took six days for it to go from uterine contractions to proper labour. The consultant encouraged her to go for a vaginal delivery after caesarean and told her that having an epidural was 'like a nice warm duvet, and it was. It was the most relaxed I'd been in a week . . . I think I would have been able to cope with twelve or fifteen hours of work, but I can't cope with six or seven days. I was gone at that stage.' After four hours she was ten centimetres dilated. The epidural meant she didn't even notice the progression, and her baby was born with minimal tearing and only one stitch. 'I felt fantastic afterwards.'

Emma, Age 44, Kildare

Emma had two vaginal deliveries after a caesarean. They were very difficult births. Her second baby was very heavy, and was distressed after the birth. They thought they were losing him at one point. 'I cried for days afterwards. I was in shock, it was awful. I was so delighted to have him, but it was awful. People don't talk about it.' On her third baby, she asked for all the drugs available. Unfortunately the birth was progressing quickly and it was too late to get an epidural or pethidine. 'It was barbaric. It was like an out-of-body experience. If I was going again I would have a section. It was dreadful. I didn't know where I was. I was screaming.' She ended up with no pain relief. She felt she couldn't even think about this lovely baby who was coming.

Andrea, Age 38, Dublin

Andrea's second baby was a VBAC. The birth went like clockwork: 'It was brilliant.' Her waters broke at home. She remembers thinking there was no way she could be only two centimetres dilated as she had been in so much pain, but once the midwife checked her, she was indeed only two centimetres dilated. But then her labour proceeded very quickly. 'Within two hours of getting into the birthing room I was fully dilated.' She thought it was going to take hours and hours. She assumed she would get pain relief at some point but was going to hold off as was nervous about slowing labour down. She also thought it was going to be a lot more painful, but in fact it was doable. She used the gas and air to help her focus on her breathing. 'It wasn't about the pain relief, it was about focusing my mind . . . It wasn't what I would describe as pain, but more like extreme discomfort.'

'I think [it would help] if people had the opportunity to go and speak openly to people who had experienced all kinds of births, not in a scaremongering kind of way, but an opportunity for them to really talk to people who had given birth . . . I hadn't really talked to anybody, I had no one-to-one conversations with somebody about what giving birth in different ways was like.'

Home Births

Laoise, Age 37, Dublin

Laoise's second baby was born at home. 'I got hot-water bottles, a TENS machine, homeopathy and a lot of kindness and small interventions early.' Her experience of the home birth was very positive. It was a very straightforward home birth, including lying down in a darkened room with her partner as he helped her through the contractions. It was very calm, and the water in the birthing pool gave amazing pain relief. Having a good midwife who knew her made all the difference to the birthing experience.

Marie, Age 49, Dublin

Marie decided on a home birth for her second baby, having had a negative experience in hospital on her first. Although it was still very, very painful, she found the pain more manageable. The subdued lighting and calm atmosphere at home made all the difference. 'I can definitely say by comparison to the first, it was totally different. It's still very, very painful . . . That did override everything . . . I can't look back and say that it was a beautiful birth in the way some people can. I didn't really sense, that it was beautiful – it was very painful, for a long time too.' She remembers delivering the placenta being quite painful too, and that surprised her.

The Dad's Point of View

Paul, Age 36, Dublin

Paul's first baby was born by planned caesarean, as their baby was breech. Both parents had been very nervous about the prospect of a natural birth and were, in fact, somewhat relieved when that decision was taken out of their hands. He is very squeamish and had thought that a caesarean would be the lesser of two evils. 'But I really, really didn't enjoy the birth experience at all . . . I was just sitting there on a stool holding my wife's hand and I was aware that she was in discomfort. It took a long time to take the baby out . . . It was a hot room, you're anxious, stressed. It was a fantastic moment when she was born but I was really not feeling great.' He didn't find it to be a memorable experience, in fact he felt disconnected from it. He ended up in a room with a hungry baby while his wife was in the recovery room, unable to feed her.

Their second baby was born naturally, and he really felt they went through it as a team. 'From the moment that her contractions began to the moment our son was born, we were together . . . I felt that I was contributing and supporting and helping . . . I found the birth experience incredibly powerful, emotional and moving in a way that a c-section just isn't . . . A c-section is an operation. With a natural birth you're seeing your partner back to their animal state. I was overcome with pride at what my wife had done.'

Barry, Age 36, Dublin

Barry found that he didn't dwell on the seriousness of the situation when his wife went into labour. He just thought about the practical stuff and tried to be as useful as he could. When it came to the birth, he didn't feel useless, as he knows some fathers can feel. He helped his wife focus on her breathing. When his first daughter was born, he felt relief more than joy. 'The one emotion was complete relief. It wasn't joy or happiness or anything like that, it was just "Thanks be to God the child is born, my wife is still here, everything seems to have gone all right." He sat in a chair with his baby while his wife was being stitched. 'The baby half-opened her eyes and sort of looked at me . . . There was a lot of activity going on in the background but I can just remember looking at her thinking 'Wow, I have a baby, this is great!' From his perspective the birth of his children was never something to be enjoyed, but something to get through, doing whatever he could do to help his wife. 'Labour is not a time where I would expect anybody to be thinking about how I feel . . . It's about the woman and the baby.'

He hated having to leave his wife and baby a few hours after the birth. 'I wasn't upset, but it felt wrong.' When he arrived home it felt weird. 'You walk in and the room was full of the pregnancy ball and all the stuff that you no longer need . . . then it hit me that things were going to change'. When he called his wife he felt frustrated because she was having to fight little battles in his absence, such as with the nurses, who were encouraging formula rather than breastfeeding. 'I should have been there but I wasn't allowed to be.' On the first day when he walked around with his baby as his wife slept, he thought 'This is lovely.' 'I had gone from being relieved to being happy.'

Terry, Age 40, Dublin

Terry felt very nervous on the birth of his baby boy. 'I didn't think too much about me, I just wanted to get the baby out safe and sound . . . I didn't mind coming second best, because to be honest with you, it's not about me.' He found it hard to watch his wife in such an inordinate amount of pain. 'I begged her to have the epidural because I wanted the pain to go away . . . I didn't want her to be in that level of distress.' He remembers the birth vividly as a very emotional and happy moment. 'I knew in that moment that this was probably the most significant moment in my life and that it was probably the most beautiful, and nothing would ever top it.' He knows that a lot of men feel traumatised by the birth, being unable to look at their wives in the same way again. He doesn't feel that at all. For him, it was overall a very positive experience that he felt very involved in. 'The birth was like a gift to me.'

Ken, Age 39, Cork

Ken was very involved with his wife's first pregnancy, learning about pressure points and shiatsu so that he could help to relieve her discomfort. However, when it came to the birth, he didn't feel welcome. 'I will freely admit I'm a bit of a control freak, but during the birth I felt I was spoken to like a child, like I was being managed. I found it quite stressful.' He would advise all parents-to-be to ensure that the dad has a clear role in the birth.

His wife was adamant that she didn't want to be induced. She went almost three weeks overdue and the birth ended up as an emergency section. Afterwards, they spoke about her decision not to be induced, and he wondered about the rights of the father, when the mother makes such a big decision about their baby. 'What if something had happened to the baby as a result of the kind of birth he had? Would I ever forgive her for making that decision on our behalf?'

Simon, Age 45, Dublin

Simon remembers feeling very protective of his wife during the births of both their children. 'It was a bit like going down a slide in one of those water parks: once the descent begins, you have no way of stopping the process until you reach the end, no matter how scary the trip turns out to be. You rationally know everybody else makes it down that slide and is OK, but it doesn't actually take away the fear for the woman, I'm sure, and certainly not for the partner . . . Just like the mum, the dad can't do anything to control the trip down that slide . . . it points out how important it is to mind each other during the process.'

When his children were born, his primary emotion was one of relief that his wife was OK. That was the most important thing. Secondly, he was relieved that his children seemed healthy and normal. 'It's very disturbing to see the person you love going through such discomfort and not being able to fix it.'

Leaving his wife in hospital after the birth of his first baby was a weird experience. He had a huge sense that life had fundamentally changed.

Contractions

When I asked the contributors what a contraction actually feels like, they all had different descriptions:

- Extreme and intense period pains (the most common answer).

- The cervix softening is like a very slow electric shock where you feel a wave of heat and tension roll up over your belly.

- A burst of emotional anguish – the kind of rush you feel when you are mourning a loved one or suffering from heartbreak, when tears come from a well deep within you that you can't control.

- Intense tightening of the abdominal and pelvic muscles.

- The inability to breathe. Like someone is shoving your head under water and until the contraction goes, you can't get your head back up again.

- The worst period pain but very much a wave up to a crescendo, and back down again.

- The opposite to throwing up (i.e. ' throwing down ').

- Pain in your whole body: an overwhelming cramp that makes you bend over and leaves you breathless.

- Pressure in the whole lower body and an intense burning pain everywhere.

- Intense squeezing all around the front and back of the abdominal and pelvic area.

- An excruciating pain somewhere deep inside that you can't access, rub or massage, somewhere near your back or your spine.

- Intense back pain – like someone rubbing a heavy rock against your tailbone.

- A very intense wave going through your body, or an intense shudder through your whole body.

Little Gems of Advice

- Babies can have their own birth plan which disregards the plan that you have made. If you remember this, you will be less stressed if you find yourself having to adapt your plan mid-labour because of changing circumstances.

- If there are certain things that you are determined to avoid (e.g. no pethidine, as it makes you nauseous), then ensure your partner is aware of these things and is prepared to fight your corner when you are mid-labour.

- At a minimum, learn how to breathe properly during labour. It can make all the difference.

- Make sure to explore all your options with your midwife or consultant if you feel that induction is being suggested prematurely.

- Induction can be much more intense than normal labour; consider an epidural if you are induced.

- The crowning of the baby's head can be quite painful; consider learning to do perineal massage as it could help with the pain and with tearing, especially for first-time mothers.

- Having a bowel movement, passing urine and vomiting during labour is quite common: don't let it shock you (the midwives have seen it all before).

- There could be other doctors/nurses/students in the delivery suite with you – if you don't want any students there, you need to be very clear about it beforehand and get your partner to back you up.

- If you are very nervous about childbirth, consider having a doula or being part of a midwife-led plan where you have the chance to build a relationship with someone who will be with you during the birth.

- During labour, try to have mini-goals to help you through the next contraction or the next half-hour rather than feeling overwhelmed at what might be coming: you don't have any way of knowing how long it's going to last or how it will go, so take it one step at a time.

- Explore the option of relaxation CDs or hypno-birthing CDs. Many of the women interviewed found them useful.

- Don't feel guilty about getting an epidural if you had planned a labour without pain relief – labour is hard work.

- Keep in mind that if you have a caesarean section, you may be limited after the birth with regards to seeing and holding your baby: if you know this going in, it might make it easier afterwards.

- Try to talk to people who have experienced lots of different types of births, especially people who will speak openly about their experiences.

- Most of the contributors agree that labour is extremely painful, so don't be disappointed in yourself or your body if you feel a sense of shock or upset afterwards.

2.
Your Body Post Birth

It's hard to imagine, until you're well into your pregnancy, what effect being pregnant will have on your body. Similarly, after childbirth, many mothers can be disappointed when they realise that childbirth and breastfeeding have left a permanent stamp on, or in, their bodies. The temporary ones range from haemorrhoids to red facial spots after pushing during childbirth. The permanent ones, on the other hand, can be shocking, whether they be stretchmarks, an altered body shape or bladder problems.

I have divided these mothers' stories into post-vaginal delivery and post-caesarean delivery sections, as the immediate physical effects after the birth can be quite different.

Post Vaginal Delivery

Kate, Age 38, Dublin

The day after the birth of my first baby, I wanted to see what damage had been done to my body. It reminded me of the opening of a volcano, with hugely swollen edges and this cavernous space . . . It's no wonder most women don't even want to look. I was relieved that I had spoken to a close friend about it before so I knew what to expect. The swelling quickly reduced and within a few days I forgot about it and it felt fairly normal. When I came back from the hospital I felt positively svelte with the loss of the bump. Part of me missed my bump though. I know I had a baby instead, and that was great, but there was something lovely about the bump, and on top of that, a bump doesn't cry or need feeding!

The birth of baby number two was a lot different, partly because he was 10 pounds 15 ounces. I had a large episiotomy scar and enormous haemorrhoids to deal with. I couldn't sit or stand up for hours due to dizziness. Then I couldn't sit because of the pain. I fed my baby lying down for a whole week. It wasn't until ten days had passed that I could finally sit properly. I had assumed that I would bounce back physically as I did first time round. It just shows you that every birth is different. You just don't know beforehand what is going to happen. Breastfeeding went well this time and at three months post birth, I was delighted to find I was a stone lighter than when I got pregnant.

Kerry, Age 37, Dublin

Kerry hadn't thought of what her body would be like after birth, focusing more on getting through labour. 'The pain of stitches was a big shock, and how tender everything was down there . . . Everything was sore, peeing really stung . . . The first time I went to the toilet for number two, I thought I was having another baby. Everything feels so loose . . . It felt like my body had been taken over for another purpose, which it had of course, and I hadn't put any thought into how that would feel.' After the first week it improved greatly.

Elaine, Age 29, Dublin

A normally slim Elaine had put on four stone during her pregnancy, and towards the end retained a lot of water. She couldn't fit back in to her maternity clothes after the birth, and went home in her pyjamas. It upset her greatly that visitors would be coming to meet her baby and she would be in her pyjamas. Two days after her return from hospital, she had to go and buy some bigger clothes. She went for a post-pregnancy massage and the water fell away within hours allowing her to fit back in to her maternity clothes. Walking was tough for a few days after the birth. She found she was really achy for about three weeks, and then it started to ease and the aching was gone by week four.

Roisín, Age 38, Belfast

Roisín was very happy that she was so physically well after the birth of her two children in the USA. She was able to sit cross-legged only a few hours after the births, and she had no stitches. She was unusual in that she lost a lot of weight while she was pregnant with her first baby and continued to lose a little more because she was combination-feeding (both by breast and by formula). She continued to lose weight when she breastfed her second baby. Being pregnant caused her to experience nausea and fatigue from eating anything more than small portions of food. This didn't disappear until well after the birth of her second child.

Jenny, Age 35, Dublin

As Jenny was part of a midwife-led pregnancy process, a midwife came to the house to check the stitches after her episiotomy. She hadn't dared to check herself. 'You don't want to look yourself. It took me a good few weeks to have the courage to look, and when I did I thought "Oh that's not so bad!"' It struck her after the birth that society focuses too much on youth and the beauty of the female form and not enough on the amazing feat the female body performs during childbirth: a true miracle of nature.

Sara, Age 39, Dublin

Having suffered from awful constipation during pregnancy, Sara was thrilled to be 'pooing like a rock star' after the birth. She had problems all her life with constipation and it seems that childbirth has cured her of this. She had no stitches and no tearing, and felt great afterwards, apart from some fissures, which subsequently healed.

Ruth, Age 36, Kildare

Ruth was very nervous the first time she went to the loo after her first birth. 'You're afraid to wash yourself, wipe yourself . . . I was terrified.' She wasn't allowed to leave the hospital until she had a bowel movement, which was fine in the end.

Cathy, Age 30, Dublin

The healing of the episiotomy hurt a lot more than she thought it would. In fact, she found the actual episiotomy and stitching pretty painful too. She didn't have a poo for seven days. After six weeks she still felt sore and bled for a long time. It stopped eventually: she just had to keep the area clean. 'It sounds worse than it was. You just had to get on with it.'

Mary, Age 32, Tipperary

Mary remembers not being able to walk very well after the birth. 'I felt like my hips had separated and I still have trouble with my hips.' They gave her a brace for a few weeks to help with the recovery. She didn't want to look at her vagina to see what it looked like, but when she first checked her scar in the shower she was quite shocked. 'It was really long and it went up towards my back passage. I didn't expect that. It had healed really well so it was grand.' She was nervous about her first visits to the loo, but she said it went absolutely fine. Because a bowel movement involves pushing the same way that you do when giving birth, 'I was nervous about stitches breaking, I didn't want to put any pressure down there', but it went fine. She took some supplements (not a laxative) from the health shop to help everything to move.

Laoise, Age 37, Dublin

Laoise hadn't expected the haemorrhoids which she noticed the day after the birth of her second child. It took about four days for them to calm down after she treated them homoeopathically and stayed in bed. 'I used to get a pain in my pelvis for a number of weeks afterwards, but I was overdoing it. Everything was a bit looser down south and if I was running, I had to work on my pelvic floor so I wouldn't pee. Everything is perfect now. It probably lasted up to twelve months.' She did some things she considers a bit stupid in retrospect, like continuing to lift the baby seat in and out of the car as if she had not just had a second baby. Looking back, she knows she could really have hurt her back in those early months.

Sinead, Age 37, Cork

On her second birth, Sinead was told to hold her breath to push, and despite only having to push five times to get the baby out, she was surprised by the red dots that appeared on her face from pushing. These faded after a few days. Physically, she noticed a big difference between the effects of a vaginal delivery and her previous caesarean. 'I was having a shower after a few hours. I felt like getting dressed and going home; I felt amazing.'

Astrid, Age 39, Germany/Dublin

Astrid was surprised by how injured and vulnerable she was after giving birth. Her midwife gave her some good advice with regards to her physical state after childbirth: 'Maybe don't look today, but maybe in the next couple of days, take a mirror and see what it looks like, or maybe feel it first.' On her first child, she didn't leave her home for two weeks as she felt this was necessary as part of her recovery. The initial healing after having stitches only took a couple of weeks, but the physical effects of breastfeeding were ongoing and she had to just accept it.

Megan, Age 40, Dublin

From the day of the birth of her son, Megan had problems with bladder control. She found herself rushing from the hospital bed to the toilet and had to restrict her water intake. She was told that things would get better. Three years later, bladder control is still a problem, and she needs to wear a sanitary towel all the time. It has been really upsetting for her. She is now seeing an expert in this area, who told her that her muscles are actually too tight and don't release easily. The physiotherapist at the hospital had taught her to tighten but never to release. 'If I have to walk far to a meeting, I have to go to the toilet first. I'm very limited.' She wonders if this is because her baby was big and she was tightening her muscles a lot to hold it, but she doesn't really know what the cause was. She says an operation could help to put this right once she has finished having children.

Megan got back into shape quicker than she thought. The breastfeeding went well, and she thinks that this has contributed to her being even thinner than she was before getting pregnant. 'My tummy is a bit flabbier than I thought it would be.'

Sarah, Age 37, Cork/London

After the birth of Sarah's first baby, it took about six weeks before the swelling went down, and it was about ten days before she could really walk properly. In the days following the births, she found the pain when going to the loo difficult to deal with and she had to move gingerly when moving from a seated to a standing position. She remembers passing large clots after her first child, but her sister-in-law was there and she reassured her that they were normal. She feels it's really important to have someone you can ask about these things.

On her second baby, she was in hospital for ten days as the baby was in special care. Despite being exhausted leaving the hospital from the constant expressing of milk and worry about her baby, physically her body had recovered from childbirth. 'I do remember being physically perfect by the time I left the hospital because I wasn't walking more than fifty yards from my ward down to the special care unit . . . you could really see the benefits of staying with your baby in the house.' On her third baby she ended up having no choice but to go on a flight after ten days due to a family emergency. 'I ended up being really ill . . . I was overdoing it.'

Rachel, Age 41, Dublin

Rachel had a very positive experience of pregnancy, birth and the early months of motherhood. However, it took longer than she expected to feel physically back to normal. 'It took me almost a year to physically feel right in myself. I didn't realise it at the time but afterwards I felt like something clicked and I was back to myself.'

Yvonne, Age 40, Dublin

On her first child, Yvonne didn't expect the amount of bleeding she experienced after childbirth, and remembers asking her mother why they had to pack pads in the hospital bag. Also, she had expected that she would lose a lot of her weight after giving birth. Before her second baby she was a size ten, so she brought a size twelve pyjamas to hospital, thinking they would fit after the birth. In fact, she was a size sixteen post birth. After her first shower, when the pyjamas wouldn't fit her, 'The midwife started laughing and I cried my eyes out . . . I didn't know that you wear maternity clothes after you have your baby.'

Tracey, Age 38, Roscommon

Tracey was shocked by the birth of her first baby girl and spent the whole of the following day reliving it. 'I was very, very sore. I had to sit on a cushion to try to sit and feed her. I found out afterwards that they had cut me up near my clitoris and never told me . . . I really didn't realise till way down the line that it had been done. It was fine if it had to be done . . . but they could at least have told me.'

After her second baby she had some pain, but took a lot more pain relief as well as arnica and some more natural topical remedies, which helped.

Kathleen, Age 38, Donegal

After the birth of her first baby, it took Kathleen nearly a year before she felt that her body was back to normal. 'I kept getting them to check me, to see if it was normal. It was such a mess; I had so many stitches.' On her second baby she insisted that the person stitching her was very experienced. It is so important that you are stitched up properly afterwards. On her first walk down to the shop with her baby, after a week, 'I had to buy myself a bottle of Lucozade to get me back, I was so drained . . . I was that dizzy.'

Anna, Age 37, Dublin

Anna had hyperemesis on both her pregnancies, which meant awful sickness throughout the entire pregnancy. 'The minute the babies were born, the hyperemesis stopped, so I stopped puking.' She had an episiotomy on her first and didn't heal well: 'nobody told me I was going to bleed for six weeks.' She had awful lower back pain after birth and it took a long time to heal. She tore on her second baby, but was told by the midwives that she didn't need to be stitched as it would heal itself, and it did.

Gemma, Age 40, Dublin

After her firstborn, Gemma felt physically back to herself after seven months (post caesarean), but three months after her second-born (vaginal delivery).

Ella, Age 45, Dublin

'I remember looking at my tummy and it was like a giant dough roll and rather grey, as if all the blood had been drained from it . . . I didn't feel like it would ever tighten up again . . . but actually when I started feeding I got pains like bad period pains. That was actually the womb contracting.'

Fionnuala, Age 40, Dublin

Fionnuala reluctantly had an episiotomy during the birth of her son. It took about six weeks to heal and she found it quite painful. Something she didn't expect afterwards was that 'I used to sweat all the time. It went on for months, I think it was hormonal . . . I don't know whether that was because I was breastfeeding.'

Suzy, Age 36, Dublin

When she was being stitched up, Suzy remembers saying to her consultant: 'This is the most important part of the entire day.' She was really worried about sex after childbirth. She remembers how relaxed she became about people looking at her vagina after days of various medics checking her stitches. 'Now I know why my mother strips off her swimming togs in a communal dressing room as if she doesn't even see the other people in the room.' She felt like a twelve-year-old wearing those enormous sanitary towels that they give you in hospital – surely, she thought, we have advanced past this!

She was very grateful that she had been told by a close friend that the bump doesn't always go down after childbirth. Her stomach was still quite big afterwards.

Deirdre, Age 40, Dublin

Deirdre was surprised by some of the physical effects of the birth after delivering her first baby, a boy. She had needed a manual extraction of the placenta as the cord had snapped during delivery, so was quite tender anyway. 'It was a week before I did a poo. It was like delivering the child all over again. I had psychologically built it up into this thing in my head . . . I think because I had had the manual extraction I was quite delicate and sore and that made things worse, but I really remember that.' On a more positive note, she walked around feeling like a model after losing the bump.

Heather, Age 39, Dublin

Heather walked like John Wayne for weeks after her baby was born. The hospital she was in was so crowded and the bathroom so far away that she remembers her bathroom visits vividly. 'The bleeding was so bad she gave me one of those sheets that they put under you when they break your waters. The midwife told me to stick it between my legs and I had to waddle to the loo in front of women and their husbands . . . I swear I must have been dripping blood . . . I felt so humiliated . . . apart from the pain.'

It was about five weeks before getting up from the couch or going up the stairs wasn't painful; she feels that this is because her baby was stuck at crowning stage for over an hour.

Andrea, Age 38, Dublin

Andrea didn't expect to be traumatised by her second baby's birth, which was a vaginal birth. She had a caesarean first time round. A week after the vaginal delivery, when the painkillers ran out, 'it hit me like a freight train . . . I just wasn't expecting it . . . I felt like my insides were about to fall out and I felt like that for about two months before I went to a doctor . . . I didn't know how I was supposed to feel.' It turned out she had a significant infection that she had been ignoring, as she has a very high pain threshold. For her, recovery wasn't easier after vaginal delivery. It was different, but not easier.

Isobel, Age 39, Dublin

Isobel remembers looking at her vagina with a mirror as she had so many stitches and was worried about getting an infection. 'I can still see the image, it was still quite open . . . I could nearly see the whole way in!' She wasn't prepared for the smell of blood and felt like people could smell it from her no matter how much she washed. She bled for three months. 'It's really hard to look after yourself. You're changing your baby's nappies, you're changing your own pads, you're changing your breast pads. I probably wasn't looking after myself properly.' She got bad thrush, which needed treatment. On top of all that, she had a problem with 'over-healing' and needed a minor procedure to remove the over-healing skin, which continued to bleed. 'Nobody tells you that your boobs are going to become engorged, that you will bleed for over six weeks. Also you're left with a basketball tummy; it doesn't automatically disappear.' She still looked pregnant a few weeks later. 'I was in maternity clothes for at least six weeks after my first pregnancy and three months after my second.'

Marie, Age 49, Dublin

Marie was surprised by the physical discomfort after the births of her two children. She found it hard to sit up comfortably in bed. 'That then has a knock-on effect on breastfeeding . . . as it was uncomfortable even sitting.' Looking back, she wishes she had been fitter physically before she had her children and wonders would that have made a difference to her recovery.

Helena, Age 33, Dublin

The day after the birth 'I was in bits . . . I felt so swollen, I couldn't walk . . . I thought the pain afterwards was worse than the labour pain.' The next day she was much improved and when she left the hospital she walked out unaided and felt a lot better, although the stitch she had was still a bit uncomfortable. That also healed up quickly once she got home.

Post Caesarean

Deborah, Age 37, Dublin

Deborah couldn't believe how big her stomach was after her caesarean section. It went down rapidly, as people kept telling her, but it surprised her. She had secretly hoped for a bit of a tummy tuck during the operation. The wound wasn't painful, but no one prepared her for the loss of sensation around the wound, which was still there eight months later.

Barbara, Age 32, Dublin

Barbara felt OK about her body after the birth of her twins by caesarean section. She felt really light, having felt huge during the pregnancy. However, 'the stretch marks were horrendous.' Two years later they are still there but look much better than they used to. 'Initially I had thought, oh God, are they always going to look this bad . . . Could I ever dream about wearing a bikini again . . . But now I'm like, yeah, so what, they are a lot paler than they were, they don't look half as bad as they used to.' She was surprised at how big her tummy was afterwards and believes that a lot of the time, it's not about weight loss but toning, and it takes time.

As for the section scar, 'it's really not that bad. In the early days you're really afraid that it'll get infected or something will happen to it, but provided you take relatively good care of it, it's not so bad.' After the birth, she was surprised that it was off-centre, and not a straight line across the middle. Two years on, she still notices the scar but doesn't fixate on it any more. 'There's nothing you can do about it, you just have to accept it. What strikes her now is that 'every time you don't have your clothes on . . . or every time you go to have sex . . . it's a mark that you've had a baby. You don't look like someone that doesn't have one . . . It's like a tattoo.'

Alison, Age 38, Kildare/San Francisco

Alison was surprised by how big her stomach still was after her caesarean section, 'I felt like I was still nine months pregnant; I didn't "deflate" quickly.'

Ella, Age 45, Dublin

Ella had her twins by caesarean section, and that was a totally different experience afterwards when compared with the birth of her first baby, by vaginal delivery. 'It was very painful . . . you can't get out of bed, you can't hold your baby, you can't go to the toilet, you have a bladder bag, you can't even really sit up in bed because the weight of your arms and upper body hurts your tummy muscles.' She didn't like that she couldn't pick up the babies and the nurses were busy. 'I was lucky to have two live babies, and the safest way to get them out was by caesarean . . . but it certainly isn't the easiest option because you've got the recovery as well for six to ten weeks afterwards.'

Emma, Age 33, Dublin

Emma's scar healed quite well after her first caesarean. She was out and about walking at two weeks and felt good, physically.

Rebecca, Age 41, Kilkenny

Rebecca remembers doing very little when she got home. 'There was a lot of sitting on the couch, and having stuff brought to me as I fed my son.' She remembers after five days going for a walk outside: 'I found that physically difficult. I was excited that I could do it, but I had to take it easy.' She also felt emotionally vulnerable. She was surprised that her tummy stayed quite big and she still looked pregnant. 'It went from that lovely hard bump to that empty saggy tummy . . . It took a while for that to go for me . . . I remember being disgusted at being left with that empty sagginess; I wasn't expecting that.' Another thing she wasn't prepared for was the new experience of piles (haemorrhoids) after childbirth. She had them for weeks and found it difficult to deal with the pain on top of everything else. She would advise new mums to be prepared for this possibility and watch their diets to avoid constipation.

Patricia, Age 35, Dublin

Patricia had never had her physical freedom curtailed like she did after her caesarean section. 'This was the first time I'd ever had six to eight weeks where I couldn't bend, I couldn't get in and out of bed easily. I was moving like an unwell ninety-year-old. That was a bit of a shock.' Her scar healed well after the first baby and she had a small infection on the second. She was surprised by the lack of information about how to manage after a caesarean. 'I was literally told don't lift anything heavier than your baby and take it easy, and given a little blue leaflet . . . but that doesn't actually tell you enough.' She had to call her consultant to see if she could go for a walk and he told her she could, but not up and down hills. There's no way she could have known that without calling him. She felt unsure about what she could and couldn't do, as she felt a pull on the stitches even when washing her hair in the shower. 'There was no real guide.'

Sinead, Age 37, Cork

After having a caesarean on her first baby, Sinead was 'totally shell-shocked.' She kept asking the doctor questions about why she still had a huge stomach. The suppositories she had been given for pain relief made her a little disoriented. She came off those and felt more pain, but more sane. 'I felt like my body was broken.' Her friend had a planned caesarean due to a breech baby, at the same time, in the same hospital. Although she had exactly the same surgery, 'she wasn't having the same problems that I was having, either mentally or physically. She was a lot happier . . . She was walking around.' She wonders if that was because, unlike her, her friend was mentally prepared for the caesarean.

Julianne, Age 39, Dublin

Julianne didn't find the caesarean painful afterwards. She thinks maybe it's because she is medically trained, that she 'took the pain relief exactly as prescribed and I didn't try to be brave, and that's my advice to anyone who has a caesarean: just take the drugs as prescribed.' She also advises that you ask for the prescription in plenty of time before you leave and have it when you're leaving so that you can get the drugs on the way home. She was shocked however by the muscle pain she felt in her back after the birth, for up to nine months.

Martha, Age 40, Wicklow

Martha felt she looked well when she was pregnant: she didn't put on much weight and was very fit physically. After her caesarean section, it took a long time for her stomach to go down, and she hated the overhang that was left from the scar initially. Since she had her son, she hasn't felt confident about how she looks. 'Nearly two years on from having him, I don't look at myself and see that I'm attractive any more . . . Even though logically I know that I'm not a whole lot heavier than I was, I feel a lot heavier . . . I feel like I'm a bit dragged and tired looking.' She doesn't have the time now to spend on herself and didn't get to the hairdressers for a year. 'I don't recognise the person I am any more.'

Andrea, Age 38, Dublin

Andrea's first baby was born by caesarean, and she had expected the recovery to be physically more traumatic than it was. She knows that she should have taken it easier not only in the weeks after the birth, but in the months to follow. During her whole maternity leave and even afterwards, she believed that 'to be a perfect mother, you have to be a perfect housewife as well . . . I was cooking, cleaning, washing. You need to give yourself a break . . . You are there to look after a child.' She found that she was pushing herself too hard, entertaining people who came to visit. She didn't do that on her second child.

Little Gems of Advice

- Most women find they still have a considerable tummy after childbirth. You could be wearing your maternity clothes for a few weeks or months after your baby arrives.

- Your body has been through a lot whether you had a vaginal delivery or a caesarean. Be kind to it and give it time to heal, time for the weight to go. Many people say it takes a year to feel back to normal physically.

- The first time you have a bowel movement can be a bit scary as the pushing sensation is similar to when you had to push your baby out (albeit much milder and usually without the pain). The anticipation of it can be worse than the actual movement itself. It can take several days, or even a week, before you have a bowel movement.

- You might be nervous about the first time you pass urine. It can sting a bit if you have had stitches, but usually it's not as bad as you think it's going to be.

- You may bleed for several weeks or even two months or more, the first few weeks usually being the heaviest. Everyone is different. There may be clots in the blood. If you're worried about their size or frequency, talk to your public health nurse or GP.

- After childbirth, don't be surprised if you have some (usually temporary) physical side effects like haemorrhoids, bloodshot eyes and small red spots on your face from pushing.

- If you do have haemorrhoids, watch your diet to avoid constipation, as that will aggravate them.

- Don't be scared by how the entrance to your vagina might look after childbirth. After a few days, it usually looks and feels more normal.

- When doing your Kegel exercises (exercises performed to strengthen the pelvic floor muscles), learning to release your muscles is just as important as learning to tighten them.

- If you have had a caesarean, don't be surprised if you find a loss of sensation around the scar that can last several months or more.

- Women who have a caesarean section have very different experiences about the length of time it takes to recover. Listen to your own body and its limitations rather than expecting to be better after a certain number of weeks.

- Don't make life harder for yourself by being slow to take your prescribed pain relief in the initial days after the birth. Take the medicines regularly to begin with.

- Don't overdo it when it comes to entertaining people at home after the birth. Give yourself a break.

- You don't need to be Super-mum or Housewife of the Year. You need to focus on getting well and minding your baby; your body has been through a lot.

3.
Mum & Baby's First Days

The first few days after a baby arrives can be an intense time. Hormones and emotions are all over the place and are often compounded by tiredness and physical exhaustion. Most of us have major expectations for the joy and elation we will experience when our baby arrives, having looked forward to it for so long. Thankfully we usually experience that to some degree, but it's often joined by anxiety, heightened emotions and the overwhelming realisation that our lives have changed dramatically forever.

Kate, Age 38, Dublin

Despite having several nights in a private room in hospital after the birth of my first baby, I found it very noisy and felt that there was very little privacy, as people were in and out of my room all the time. I don't think there is any perfect solution for where to spend those first few days after the birth: private rooms or public wards, home or hospital, it depends on the person and their individual needs. I felt very vulnerable on my own at night when my husband went home. I was watching the clock in the morning, waiting for him to come back in. I had little or no sleep, as I was so shocked after the birth that I couldn't sleep properly. I wish I had been home in my own bed with him. Although I felt very protective of my baby in those early days, all of my feelings were overshadowed by the shock of childbirth and exhaustion. It took weeks for that to lift.

On my second baby, I came home the following day. Although I felt a little vulnerable, as I was physically weak after a difficult birth, I felt much happier being at home than in the ward that I had been in on the first night. At least I could sleep with earplugs in, knowing my husband was able to look after the baby. I always had someone there to help, unlike at the hospital.

Martha, Age 40, Wicklow

Because she had her own room in the hospital, Martha felt quite isolated. The midwives and nurses were amazing when they did come, but they were overstretched and didn't have a lot of time. She loved her son 'but I had no idea who he was. I found that quite disconcerting . . . My instinct was so strong to protect him.' She didn't feel love and a bond the minute she looked at him, the way other women say they do. 'I felt odd about it. Was I supposed to look at this child and feel that? But I did look at him and think: Oh my God, I made this little being.'

Emma, Age 44, Kildare

Emma didn't know if she would ever have children. She remembers coming home with her first baby. 'I cried the whole way home. They had let me out with this baby. That was it now, there was no help. I had three hours' sleep in five days, as I was breast-feeding him and fed him day and night.' She was nervous and overjoyed at the same time. 'I hadn't a clue. But it was lovely, just him and me. I never saw so much daytime TV.'

Barbara, Age 32, Dublin

Barbara's twin babies were born by an unplanned caesarean section. They were taken to ICU immediately and she didn't see them again that day, having held them only briefly. When she saw them the next morning, it was a strange experience. 'I couldn't hold them or touch them, they were in their incubators . . . It was really bizarre because I went from being a normal person the day before, to being in a wheelchair, sitting beside these incubators, looking at these babies who were supposed to be my babies. They could have wheeled me over to any incubator and said 'These are your kids' . . . It was strange.'

Patricia, Age 35, Dublin

Patricia certainly had that happy glow of having a new baby. However, she was shocked by what she had gone through. She had a very difficult labour that ended in a caesarean section. 'I remember coming home to the house . . . As soon as I got in the door of the house I just cried and cried and cried . . . I couldn't believe I was home again after all I'd been through . . . It felt like I'd come out the other side of the tunnel.' The second night after her first baby was born, exhausted after almost seven nights with little or no sleep, Patricia remembers her son opening his eyes and staring at her, frowning. 'I remember thinking he doesn't like me . . . I remember getting a fright.' She believes it was pure exhaustion that gave her those thoughts.

Patricia feels that it's important to know that not everyone is gazing at their baby with love and admiration, that lots of people are scared stiff. 'Do not freak out if you suddenly think, I'm not enjoying this.' Even though she had read about the 'baby blues', she didn't recognise that this was what it was, when she was in the middle of it.

Rebecca, Age 41, Kilkenny

Rebecca was quite high on morphine after her firstborn was delivered via caesarean section. She didn't like the effect it had on her mind and so accepted less pain relief after the birth of her second baby (also by caesarean). 'For the first twelve hours or so it was really, really painful across my middle, and trying to sit up was very difficult . . . The intensity of the pain did ease but it was hard to get around.'

Laoise, Age 37 Dublin

Laoise had laboured at home, intending to deliver there, but had to go to hospital for the birth. She came home very soon afterwards. The midwife who was at home had tidied everything. 'One thing about a home birth is that you are on medical advice to do nothing . . . I was instructed to stay in bed for two weeks. It was medically indicated that I stay in bed: it's part of the home-birth after care.' Laoise called it her 'babymoon'. It really clicked with her more on her second baby that 'this is all so temporary, it won't last', so she spent as much time in bed with the baby as she could.

On her first, she thought she would get her life back to normal very quickly, and put herself under pressure to be on time for things and to go out a lot. It took her a while to understand how ridiculous that was.

Rachel, Age 41, Dublin

The person Rachel wanted to see the most in the days after giving birth, while still in hospital, was her mother. 'I was almost watching out to see if she'd stick her head around the curtain. I felt like a child again the day or two after I had my daughter . . . When we feel like a child we want our Mammies. I also wanted her to see my beautiful daughter. My mother died when I was fourteen, so she was never going to stick her head around the curtain.'

Kathleen, Age 38, Dublin

She was happy enough with the care she received in the hospital after giving birth to her first baby, but she does remember having to wait a long time for pain relief. She was in a lot of pain. Despite having already been examined, another midwife checked her and told her she had what was called a 'proud stitch'. This is where a bit of skin has been stitched into a stitch; this can be extremely sore. She would advise any new mother not to leave the hospital without a prescription for pain relief.

Her daughter was placed in the special care unit after she was born, as a precaution. 'For me that was quite good, because I slept for the first night. They came in and asked me on the second night if I wanted to keep her with me . . . I stupidly said yes . . . In hindsight I should have told them to keep her and bring her to me to be fed, because I would have slept better.'

Michelle, Age 30, Dublin

After her baby girl was born by caesarean, Michelle felt she was in shock, but she was euphoric at the same time. 'They took the baby away from me because I had a section. I was wheeled in to the recovery room; I didn't know where she was. She was with my husband, but I didn't know that.' Unfortunately, the staff all changed over at that point, so it took quite a while for someone to let her know where the baby was. 'Once I knew where they were, I was fine. I was so out of it, but I had a bit of a snooze at that stage.' Michelle feels that for the first twenty-four hours after having a section, you wonder if you'll ever be normal again. Trying to sit up was so difficult. People had to give her the baby from the cot beside her. 'It's really hard but you're so happy, it's crazy.' The first walk to the shower was horrific: she was shuffling, along dragging her urinary catheter bag beside her. Taking her clothes off was really difficult, so she sat down and 'had a little cry' in the shower. Forty-eight hours later she noticed a huge improvement. She kept telling other mothers she saw in the corridors crying after a caesarean that things would improve. A caesarean might make the birth easy 'but the recovery is really tough.'

Anna, Age 37, Dublin

After her first baby, Anna stayed in hospital. She didn't sleep, her baby was crying and she didn't know if she was feeding her properly. 'I was absolutely distraught and tired . . . I hadn't slept for three days.' 'After my second child was born, I went home straight away. I felt like it had been so easy, I could do that again tomorrow.' She didn't feel awful tiredness once she had got home and was able to get some sleep.

Gemma, Age 40, Dublin

Gemma's second son was born with Down syndrome. He was born early and she initially thought this explained the puffy look around his eyes. She asked if it was normal and the consultant looked at her with eyes that told her it wasn't. She knew then that he had Down syndrome. 'It was like being kicked in the stomach, and surreal. It's like they're telling someone else . . . It made it difficult just to be with him as a tiny baby.' They decided not to think about the fact that he had Down syndrome straight away but to focus on enjoying him. 'It's paradoxical: you have this beautiful tiny baby, but you also are looking at something you don't have a lot of knowledge about . . . Fortunately I was in good physical condition to look after him.' Her parents were upset for them, but both their parents have been wonderful. 'It's funny who we have experienced as being supportive and not supportive . . . Maybe it's very close to the bone for some people.' The care they received in hospital after his birth was amazing. 'We were surrounded by kindness and caring.'

Emma, Age 33, Dublin

Emma remembers the baby blues coming in after a couple of days. She remembers how it felt when her husband came in and straight away asked how the baby was. 'I thought, "I've just had major abdominal surgery! That baby is fine!" Of course I cared about how the baby was, but it was really difficult, that idea that you don't really matter any more.'

Andrea, Age 38, Dublin

Andrea's first night at hospital was a bit of a blur, as she was on morphine. What surprised her on her third night was what happened to her body when her milk came in. 'Nobody had really explained to me how it would happen. Suddenly I felt like I had these bricks strapped on to me. It's so painful. I didn't realise that it meant my milk had come in.' The ward was noisy. She had very little sleep at this stage and was starting to feel a bit overwhelmed. 'I woke up and I was absolutely drenched.' She thought she was sweating, and changed her nightdress, but an hour later she was drenched again. 'I realise in retrospect that it was my milk, but again nobody had explained that to me.'

Marie, Age 49, Dublin

After the births of both of her children, Marie stayed in bed with her babies for at least two weeks. She remembers that time very warmly. She had calm music on and that created a lovely safe atmosphere. She remembers her cousin coming up to her room to visit and saying, 'Oh, you'd want to turn up that radio and make it nice and loud because you know, get them used to it, the world's like that, it's going to be very noisy.' She didn't take her advice.

Little Gems of Advice

- If you have a caesarean section, you should be prepared for the fact that you may not see your baby much for the few hours after the birth, as you will be recovering from major abdominal surgery. Your partner will probably be the one 'holding the baby'.

- Don't worry if you don't feel a bond with your baby from day one. Lots of women find that it takes time to get to know their baby before they really feel that motherly love they've heard and read about.

- Don't be surprised if you feel completely overwhelmed when you come home from hospital: you have been through a life-changing event. Don't be afraid if you find yourself crying in that first week or so. Just have a good cry and take each day as it comes.

- Don't put pressure on yourself to get 'back to normal' in those early days, weeks and months. For most women, life has permanently changed. There will be a new 'normal' that will emerge eventually.

- Don't leave the hospital without a prescription for pain relief.

- Be prepared for when your milk comes in, usually after two or three days. It is quite a major physical change, so keep your eye out for it and get the midwives to help you manage it.

- When you get home from the hospital, create a calm, warm atmosphere for both you and the baby. You've both been through a major life event.

4.
Feeding

'Breast is best' is a phrase that is used regularly, whether it be on hospital pamphlets or television adverts or at ante-natal classes. The majority of women I interviewed agreed with this phrase and had intended to breast feed their babies. Here are some statistics about breastfeeding rates in Ireland and how we compare with other European countries:

- Rates of breastfeeding in the Republic of Ireland are low by international standards. Just over 50 percent of mothers currently initiate breastfeeding in Ireland compared to 81 percent in the UK and over 90 percent in Scandinavian states.[1]

- Only 22 percent of babies in Ireland are exclusively breastfed at three months.[2]

- Across Europe on average nine out of every ten babies born are breastfed.[3]

Although the majority of the women interviewed did breastfeed their babies, many of them did not have a positive experience, particularly at the beginning. I was struck by the lack of support they received, either to initiate or to continue breastfeeding. Most of the women I interviewed who were unable to breastfeed were hugely disappointed and felt an overwhelming sense of guilt when they made the decision to stop trying to breastfeed and moved to formula milk.

Breastfeeding

Kate, Age 38, Dublin

After a very negative experience with breastfeeding on my first baby, I was hoping that I would manage to breastfeed my second. He latched on straight away. I never once experienced soreness, cracked nipples or the like. He fed like a dream and, on a superficial note, I am skinnier than I have been in ten years! It proved to me that it wasn't my fault first time round. I didn't do anything different this time; it just worked. I had the community midwives visiting every day for a week and they were brilliant. I also had a great lactation consultant, who visited me when I came home. She helped a lot and reassured me that I was doing it 'right'. I would advise anyone to have that kind of support lined up if they really want to breastfeed.

Ella, Age 45, Dublin

Breastfeeding was really difficult on her first baby. 'I expressed for eight weeks and I just kept trying to breastfeed him and eventually he gave in and I breastfed him till he was six months . . . so it worked out in the end.' Those first eight weeks were very difficult and she had to spend time pumping and sterilising after having tried to breastfeed him. 'I was determined that it would work.' She had had to give him formula initially as he had jaundice and her milk was slow coming in, so she had no choice in the matter. 'A lactation consultant might say differently, but I think it was the right thing to do at the time.' She attended a breastfeeding group for some support while she was exclusively expressing. 'I took out my bottle and asked if anyone else was exclusively expressing, and they all looked at me like I'd brought a bottle of vodka to an AA meeting.' She just persevered with it and fed the baby when he was tired and a bit dopey and it got him used to the breastfeeding. She kept looking for help from various sources. 'My mum and husband both told me to stop breastfeeding . . . I was disappointed in both of them . . . I needed someone to tell me just to try for one more day.'

Barbara, Age 32, Dublin

Despite many hospitals in Ireland stating their preference for breastfeeding, the experience for Barbara was quite different. Having had twins, the midwives were surprised at her determination to breastfeed or express in order to feed the babies, who were in ICU. She made a big deal about it and insisted that they not be formula fed until she saw a lactation consultant. 'They obviously just thought I was a nutter, because they were twins, underweight and in ICU.' Afterwards, she saw her chart. The consultant had written 'Mum really into breastfeeding' underlined several times. She thinks that her insistence meant that she saw the lactation consultant more quickly than most people. This meant that she was prepared for the lengthy expressing routine that was to follow, once her milk came in.

She was at a really low point a couple of weeks after her boys were born and was finding the breastfeeding very hard. The lactation consultant gave her great advice. 'It's only for such a short period of time. That's what you have got to keep telling yourself. It feels like this time will never end, but you will look back and realise it was just the first three months. The time passes.' This piece of advice really helped her get through those tough weeks.

Emma, Age 44, Kildare

Emma breastfed her first baby. 'I had a fabulous latch-on in the hospital. It was like he knew that I hadn't a clue. It was like magic. I felt like Mum of the Year. That was it: we had a bond.' Breastfeeding was hard for her though. It hurt and didn't come naturally to her once she got home. She wishes she had had more help at home with breastfeeding. The local breastfeeding group wasn't very helpful. She went to another more 'purist' breastfeeding group and felt very unwelcome, as she was supplementing with formula. 'I said "But this is getting me through, getting me some sleep." But no. It was all-or-nothing for them: I was nearly kicked out.' She breastfed her second baby too and found it a bit easier. 'But then I realised, it's not the be-all-and-end-all. I didn't do the martyr on it and gave up when I was ready, after about three months.' She breastfed her third baby for five days but then stopped, as she felt her relationship with her second boy, who was still very young, was suffering. He wasn't coping well because he needed her. 'I cried for a few days but the house was much better for everybody: everybody got the attention they needed.'

Deborah, Age 37, Dublin

Deborah really wanted to breastfeed. There was little support at the hospital until she made a scene, demanding some time with the lactation consultant. Luckily she ended up with a positive experience breastfeeding her baby. She felt, however, that the tiredness of being a new mother was accentuated by breastfeeding her baby, and found it quite draining. She would advise anyone who is breastfeeding to remember that for many women, it can take a lot out of you, so take care of yourself and take it easy.

Jenny, Age 35, Dublin

Jenny had quite a positive experience breastfeeding her daughter. 'No one really explains to you what it's going to be like. I really wanted to do it and I'm very pleased that I did. It's quite painful when the milk's coming in. I hadn't really expected that.' At the breastfeeding classes in the hospital before the birth, the midwives were very pro-breastfeeding. Ironically, in the days after the birth the midwives, who were overstretched, weren't able to help much. One of the first nights, when the baby was unsettled, she was offered a bottle of formula. She said no and was glad that she did, because her baby latched on the next day. She had read that babies don't normally need a high volume of milk in the first few days. 'In the dark hours of the night when you're on your own, you need a professional to say that it's OK, that they don't need this. Instead they wanted to shove the bottle in to keep the baby quiet. That's what I felt anyway.'

When her parents came to visit at the hospital, she was very conscious that if the baby woke up she would have to breastfeed in front of her dad. 'I was really off with dad, because I was really worried that was going to happen. Now, of course I would just ask him to go out, or I would get one of those cover things.' She knows now that she just should have been honest with him and he would have been fine with it. 'Just because you're breastfeeding doesn't mean you're suddenly happy for your dad to see your boobs.'

Sara, Age 39, Dublin

Sara had a very positive experience with the community midwives at her local hospital. 'Even before I left the delivery room she had been put on my boob . . . They were showing me lots of different types of holds, because I have very big breasts . . . so I went home with all of that knowledge.' The midwives visited her at home every day and she believes that this consistent support helped her to have a positive experience of breastfeeding.

Cathy, Age 30, Dublin

Cathy was happy with how breastfeeding went. There were no problems with latching on, and she breastfed her daughter exclusively for the first three months. 'I'm very big-chested and when I was nursing at first they got insanely large, and I found nursing bras very hard to find, and that made it very uncomfortable.' She also found that because she is big-chested, it was difficult to breastfeed discreetly.

Rebecca, Age 41, Kilkenny

Breastfeeding her first baby was very difficult, and not at all what she expected. 'It hurt my nipples and my boobs were really sore filling up with milk.' Like most women, her milk didn't come in until a few days after the birth, but her babies were hungry from day one. Some of the midwives were pushing formula at this point but she really wanted to persevere. To complicate things further, three midwives were giving her conflicting advice. 'I could have done it differently maybe if I had had someone who knew what they were doing helping me.' She doesn't have positive memories of feeding in those first few days 'I remember sitting in a chair . . . One of my breasts was engorged with milk, one of the midwives had me and the other was trying to shove his mouth in to my nipple; we were both crying.' She was more relaxed on her second baby and although it was still sore, it was easier.

Laoise, Age 37, Dublin

Breastfeeding went very well for Laoise with both her babies. Her home-birth midwife stayed till 4 AM to make sure that she had her latch right and to support her. On her first birth, when she unexpectedly had to go in to the hospital after labouring at home, she was pressing the call-button, looking for help, but the midwives were so busy, they didn't come. They were nice and meant well but were overstretched and didn't have time. She thinks that the midwives at the hospital are very pro-breastfeeding, but then when mothers go home, often on day three when the milk is only coming in, things can go wrong. 'That's when the downer hormones come in . . . You turn into a nutcase on day four and then you're

sent home and told "If you don't breastfeed you're a bad mother."
It's a form of abuse if you ask me!'

Caroline, Age 35, Dublin

Caroline had a positive experience breastfeeding her baby boy.
However, she did find it very painful when he latched, and had a
lot of bleeding. She had found a great guide to breastfeeding and
this helped her, along with advice from her mum and a great midwife at the hospital. She was also very determined and feels that
she was lucky it worked out for her.

Sinead, Age 37, Cork

Sinead's first baby was born by caesarean section, which disappointed her, as she had wanted a natural delivery. On top of this,
he wouldn't breastfeed: he was three weeks overdue, very big and
extremely hungry. The midwives gave him formula, which
depressed and upset her further. They told her she could express
whatever she had and they could feed him from a bottle. She tried
to express and had no milk but had colostrum (watery pre-milk
that secretes from the breast in the first days after delivery), which
she fed him. There was conflicting advice from all the midwives at
the hospital. 'I definitely felt like they were talking the talk but not
walking the walk', promoting breastfeeding in one breath and
offering formula in the next. Between a lactation consultant and
her mum, by the time he was ten days old, 'I had weaned him off
the formula and on to the breast.' She feels it was sheer determination and stubbornness on her part, and she breastfed him for ten
months. 'I think teaching him to breastfeed saved me mentally
because I felt like I had succeeded at something and the birth felt
like a failure . . . I felt that if I couldn't manage to breastfeed him,
then my body would have failed me again . . . It helped me bond
with him; it was a massive turning point for me after he was born.'

Astrid, Age 39, Dublin

Astrid breastfed both of her babies. She found it just worked for her. Most of her friends and family had positive experiences of breastfeeding. Her first baby was born in Germany, where she had great support from the midwife at home, and could have had more of her time if needed. She does remember having early signs of mastitis and thinks that she was overdoing it. 'You need to rest . . . I wanted to visit friends; I had to move house. You should try not to pack too much in for the first two or three months.'

Megan, Age 39, Dublin

Breastfeeding went well for Megan for the first three weeks. 'Then I decided to express, and I gave myself mastitis, as I had been producing a lot of milk.' She overproduced milk and woke up at 5 AM with a really sore breast, and sweating. She went in to the hospital and saw the breastfeeding consultant, who prescribed antibiotics, which worked within twenty-four hours. She knows that if you don't deal with it properly, mastitis can be very dangerous. 'It was a really good warning, because then I was religious about it . . . I am one of a small percentage of women who produce too much milk.' Her baby fed really well, and she never had sore breasts from feeding. She puts it down to luck mostly. Looking back, Megan thinks that she should have been less strict about formula. If she had offered him a bottle more often, it would have given her a much-needed break from the breastfeeding and expressing.

Sarah, Age 37, Cork/London

Sarah breastfed her three children. She was very lucky; it went very well from the beginning. 'My only concern was that she only fed for five or six minutes . . . She was never latched on for very long.' She asked the midwife on day five if she should worry, as she had read about people feeding constantly, but the midwife observed a feed and said that things were fine and that the baby was putting on weight. All of her children ended up like that. She puts it down to luck and also to her attitude to the feeding. She was very relaxed and felt confident that it would work. 'I went to a lot of breastfeeding groups and saw people who are not so confident with themselves and worried about their baby not putting on weight . . . and falling into the trap of feeding the baby all day and all night, so your milk doesn't have a chance to replenish, and you get exhausted.'

Rachel, Age 41, Dublin

Rachel wanted to breastfeed her first baby. 'I was very clear in my head, if this doesn't work, it doesn't work. I wasn't going to be a breastfeeding martyr; I'm not going to kill myself over it.' On the second night after the birth, her baby cried for three or four hours and wasn't latching on well. The nurse suggested a bottle but Rachel worried that she wouldn't be able to breastfeed after that. She hadn't slept for two nights and the baby blues were kicking in. The ward sister came round and said: 'We are so hard on ourselves as women; there is no reason why you can't go back and try breast-feeding again if you want.' Rachel said she felt like she 'was feeding her a bottle of arsenic or something, it was upsetting her so much.' She got lots of help with breastfeeding from the midwives at the hospital, although it took her a good few days to master it, and it hurt. She breastfed her up to eleven weeks, after which she was happy to move on to formula. She really enjoyed breastfeeding and the bond it created. 'It was really powerful. You could put me down in a ditch on the side of the road while I was feeding her and I wouldn't have cared.'

Kathleen, Age 38, Donegal

Kathleen breastfed both her babies. She was happy with the

experience and had no major problems. 'I had decided that's what I was going to do. I did do a bit of research beforehand.' She learned a lot about how the system worked in the hospital. 'Someone had advised me that when you decide you want to breastfeed, be adamant you are going to breastfeed and don't take no for an answer . . . I found that if you said 'I am breastfeeding', the people who are not bothered with breastfeeding left you alone and the people who were interested in breastfeeding gave you more attention and helped you.' She found that she received conflicting advice between midwives about breastfeeding.

Suzy, Age 36, Dublin

Suzy's baby was a 'sucky baby'. The first night after he was born, her nipples were destroyed from feeding. Even the lactation consultant said that she had never seen anything like it. Suzy was advised to give him a soother but said no, because she was worried about nipple confusion. A different lactation consultant gave her the same advice. 'I said, "But Google said . . ." and she flipped at me, and rightly so, saying "Google? How do you even have access to Google?! I'm telling you right now you need to get that child a soother and that's the end of it."' She believes that was the beginning of a phase of anxiety for her. 'I think it's something particular to our generation, everything needs to be triple-checked before you make a decision on it.' Three days later, on Christmas Eve, her mother was in the only chemist open in the city looking for a soother.

She found the early feeding days so difficult. She called everyone she knew who had breastfed, asking them if it was really supposed to be this difficult. 'Of course, everybody had struggled . . . but I was looking for a licence to stop, and nobody was ever going to give that to me.' She fed him for three months and now she thinks that was a mistake. It never got easy for her. 'I had to stop going [to the breastfeeding classes] because I was like the person they couldn't fix. I was actually making them uncomfortable. I used to gag while he was feeding because he sucked so hard.' She kept going because she felt that this was the first job she had to do for him. She had read about the benefits of breastfeeding in the first three months. 'I knew medically this was better for him, so I'll do everything I have to do.' On her next baby, if it is as difficult again, she does not plan to persist as far as the three-month point.

Suzy firmly believes that some women just can't breastfeed, while another large group of women can breastfeed, but need a lot of support. 'I just needed somebody qualified to tell me to stop.' It didn't matter that her mother and her husband thought she should. 'My husband would say that I was a nightmare and not nice to live with.'

She was scared of the next feed. She even lied to her husband about how long she had fed the baby for, because she just couldn't feed him for longer than a few minutes. 'They [breastfeeding advocates] make out that formula is made from rusty nails, frogs' legs and the hair of a witch. Really it's a multi-vitamin and the child will be absolutely fine.'

Martha, Age 40, Wicklow

Martha breastfed her baby boy. She was surprised by the number of people who told her to give him a bottle and not to be so hard on herself. She really wanted to breastfeed. Her GP pointed out that she was tying herself in knots over breastfeeding and asked her why she was continuing it after ten weeks when she found it so hard. This upset her as she was determined, and felt very guilty at the thought of giving up. 'Maybe it would have been better if she had said "You don't have to do this, but I can get you help if you need it."'

Looking back, she thinks she should have been more assertive

than sitting up straight. She couldn't get proper back support with the pillows she had. She was never shown how to feed lying down. She left hospital with very bad back pain, and exhausted after several days of very little sleep.

She was determined to breastfeed in part because she was concerned she wouldn't bond with her son. When she got back from hospital, 'I had no support at all. I know there is support there and I am involved with them now, but in those early days . . . I thought I could figure it out for myself. It takes a lot before I'd ask for help.' She now knows that no matter how stupid it seems, mothers shouldn't be afraid to ask questions to help with breastfeeding. At the hospital, her son was given a bottle of formula on the second night. The midwife knew Fionnuala was trying to breastfeed and although she was pleasant and well-meaning, Fionnuala felt that her advice was full of contradictions. If she has another baby, she will be more confident to just persevere with the breastfeeding and say no to the bottle of formula.

She found that some of the breastfeeding groups were very purist and lacked flexibility. The best group she found was full of open-minded mothers who 'don't look down their nose' if you're combination-feeding. She feels it depends on the individuals involved in the groups, so new mums should go along and see what the groups are like before their baby arrives.

Deirdre, Age 40, Dublin

Deirdre exclusively breastfed her first baby for four months and combination-fed her second baby. On her first, 'I found breastfeeding brutal, to be honest, the feeling when it wasn't working, that I'm letting my child down, I'm a failure, I'm not a good mum, to the sheer drain that is on you physically . . . This child was there every two hours and he didn't sleep very well because he wasn't full.' It went a lot better on her second baby, when she combination-fed.

In the ante-natal classes the midwives were promoting breast-feeding. 'You're in the hospital, and did anyone come round to help me breastfeed? No. He screamed his way through his second night and I'm in a ward with four other people.' The nurses did come eventually and asked her if she wanted to give him a bottle of formula. It wasn't how she wanted it to be, and she was worried that she was going to be a complete failure. 'It's not the end of the world if they get a few ounces on day two from a bottle. To me it's just scaremongering to say that they'll never feed off the breast again . . . I think it's kind of wrong that women are putting other women under pressure. You're all comrades-in-arms . . . If a man was coming in doing it, we'd be giving out!'

Heather, Age 39, Dublin

Heather breastfed her baby boy. 'It is probably the most traumatic thing I have ever experienced in my life, and I have been through quite a few things. That was the most physically and emotionally painful experience . . . The reason ultimately was because he wasn't feeding properly and he kept crying for weeks and weeks.' She was told by her doctor that babies just cry. The public health nurse said that he was 'just a minx', and she should let him cry. 'Because he wasn't feeding properly, I was not getting all the milk out and ultimately ended up with mastitis and a breast abscess.' Their doctor thought the baby had reflux, but when they went back to the hospital, a midwife happened to be nearby and heard his cry and commented that his cry was a hungry cry. The midwife was right: he wasn't getting enough milk. The lactation consultant diagnosed a posterior tongue tie, which resolved itself in the end.

Her public health nurse had told her that breastfeeding hurts and that's just how it is. She agrees that yes, it can hurt, but this was pain at a level she couldn't manage, and she has quite a high pain threshold. 'I was crying every time I fed him. He was feeding around the clock and I was dreading every feed.' She feels that the emotional pressure from the hospital that 'breastfeeding is best' was huge. Her doctor was very supportive and organised for her breast abscess to be finally drained at week thirteen. 'Suddenly it didn't hurt any more.' She wanted someone to tell her that she didn't need to continue to breastfeed, that she should move on to formula. However, when the doctors at the hospital told her she was crazy to continue breastfeeding, she couldn't stop. 'I couldn't because of the guilt . . . but I'm glad I didn't stop, because in the long run, if you keep going it turns into the easiest thing in the world.' Heather believes that when you're not feeding around the clock, as you are at the beginning, it's much easier. It doesn't hurt and your body becomes more able to produce the right amount of milk for the right time. She also thinks that there's something in the breast milk, like an anti-depressant, that keeps you going through those sleepless nights. In retrospect she wishes she had availed of the services of a lactation consultant to visit her at home and help her in those early days.

Patricia, Age 35, Dublin

Patricia was happy with how the experience of breastfeeding went with both of her babies. For her first baby, she asked for a lot of help in the hospital and asked a midwife to check the latch every time she fed her baby. 'I was very determined to do it and that really helps too.' She believes that if you go into it with the attitude that you'll try it and see what happens, you will probably fail at the first hurdle, 'because . . . those early weeks are very hard.' She had done some reading on breastfeeding. She had also identified a lactation consultant, who came around and reassured her that she was doing well.

Despite the success with the feeding, she did feel overwhelmed. In the hospital, one midwife would tell her not to wake a sleeping baby, the next came in and advised her to wake him after five hours, and the midwife on the next shift told her she shouldn't let a tiny baby go more than two and a half hours without being fed. When she discussed this conflict of information with the lactation consultant a few weeks later, she told her that, in a way, they were all correct: that there is no wrong way to do it. 'But when you're vulnerable like that, you need [to hear] the party line, you don't need all this conflicting advice, and then being told either "trust your instincts" or "you decide".'

Julianne, Age 39, Dublin

Julianne breastfed both her babies. She was happy with how it went, though she was sore for the first six to eight weeks on her first baby. She doesn't believe that you're doing it wrong if it's sore: 'Sometimes it's just sore.' Her baby gained weight well. She got great advice from a breastfeeding counsellor at a class: 'If you're having a bad feed, just say to yourself, I'll get through this one and I'll see what happens at the next feed. Try not to look too far ahead.' She thinks this helped her a lot.

Andrea, Age 38, Dublin

Andrea assumed that breastfeeding would be difficult. However, on both of her babies it went brilliantly. 'I do not believe that breastfeeding is natural, therefore it comes naturally.' She knows that it takes work to get it right. She puts her success down to preparation and good luck. She went to an ante-natal breastfeeding class at the hospital, watched DVDs on breastfeeding, and read books about the science of breast milk and breastfeeding. All of this gave her great confidence about her decisions once she started feeding. 'It just happened. They both latched on from the word go. I never had sore nipples, bleeding nipples; I had none of that.'

Isobel, Age 39, Dublin

Isobel found it easy to breastfeed, and that surprised her, as she was small-chested, dispelling the myth that having small breasts means you won't be able to breastfeed. 'I was very lucky: she latched on immediately . . . I don't think it was the right thing for me psychologically though; it definitely turned me into a nutcase.' She was a nervous wreck in social situations, as she wasn't comfortable breastfeeding in public. In retrospect, she wishes she hadn't been such a purist and that she had introduced a bottle earlier. Her daughter cluster-fed from 10 PM to 1 AM every night. 'Breastfeeding isn't for everyone and I don't think it's for me, even though I've done it for both my kids.' She feels that as a breastfeeding mother you can feel really alone, as you're the only one who can do it.

She felt peer pressure from other mothers at the breastfeeding group. She would advise a new mother: 'Don't be afraid to give up, you're not a failure.' She also wishes she had been more prepared for breastfeeding in public. She was very uncomfortable with it and it made her feel stressed when she was out. If a new mum is worried about feeding in public, she would advise them: 'Do your research in advance, find out what cafés have nice comfy sofas in quiet corners . . . Don't sit in an exposed spot if you're going to be adjusting your baby or manoeuvring your boob out and latching your baby on.'

Marie, Age 49, Dublin

Marie breastfed both of her babies. Within hours of giving birth to her first baby, she got conflicting advice from various midwives. 'One midwife would come in and say, "Make sure that you breastfeed a little bit on each side and time it, and write it down", then the next one would come in and say, "What's this big list of times and things? Why are you doing it that way? No, no, just feed her whenever she needs to feed."' She would have found it helpful if that initial information had been consistent. 'I don't think it's even the job of the midwife. They are run off their feet . . . You need somebody standing beside you for a whole day.' When she got home, her friend nagged her to go to a local breastfeeding group, a resource that, in the end, helped her hugely.

She thinks that if you're interested in breastfeeding it makes sense to go to a few meetings before the birth and find a meeting that suits you so that you can get the support you need.

Ruth, Age 36, Dublin

Ruth was only nineteen years old when she had her first baby. She chose to breastfeed, and it didn't go as well as she had hoped. 'I got no support for breastfeeding . . . My mam's friends wouldn't come into the room if I was breastfeeding.' She introduced formula quite early, based on advice from other women, and very quickly her milk supply reduced. 'I didn't know about breastfeeding support . . . I didn't even know what a breast pump was.' If she had her time again, she would have asked about breastfeeding support groups and not listened to advice from people who had never breastfed.

Mary, Age 32, Tipperary

Mary exclusively breastfed her daughter for two weeks before introducing formula. She loved the feeling of breastfeeding. 'I just wanted her near, and I was so happy that I didn't have to give her anything man-made. I felt really close to her; I felt it was the best thing for her.' But as the weeks went on and her baby's appetite increased, 'I was just exhausted and I was getting emotional with it and I was so drained. I thought: I'm no good to her if I'm exhausted.' She was a bit hard on herself, and 'felt like a bit of a failure. There was a lot of guilt, and I hummed and hawed about it. I was comparing myself to everyone else. The next time I wouldn't be so hard on myself.'

Formula-Feeding

Kate, Age 38, Dublin

I really wanted to breastfeed my first baby. Despite trying for almost a week, my baby did not latch on properly, so I expressed for three weeks instead and combination-fed with formula and breast milk. I was surprised by how overwhelming I found the whole bottles and formula process. Because I was so tired, I couldn't get my head around basic things like how the steriliser worked or how to clean it. Once I introduced formula to the equation I got even more stressed. I used to get my sister to pick up trays of pre-prepared formula in disposable bottles that they give you in the hospital, because I couldn't cope with the job of mixing water and powder. It cost a small fortune. That's how messed up my head was.

Before the birth, I had a very practical approach, attending a breastfeeding class and finding a lactation consultant who would come to the house if I needed her after the birth. I told myself that if it didn't work out, it wasn't going to be a big deal. However, after the birth, when the hormones and tiredness kicked in, I was devastated that my baby wouldn't latch. I felt like I had failed my baby on my most important job, the one job that only I could do for her. Despite every midwife in the hospital pulling and dragging at me, using nipple shields, and a visit from the lactation consultant, the baby just would not latch. People tried to say helpful things like 'Keep trying, it's natural, it'll happen' but my baby was hungry and I was truly exhausted. The guilt was unbearable. I expressed for three weeks so that I wouldn't feel so guilty. Looking back, I wish that I had released myself from that guilt a lot earlier and focused on getting sleep and loving my baby. That baby is now over three years old and experiences, in general, better health than some of her breastfed friends. This isn't because she was bottle-fed. I think it's just her genes. Formula did not do her any harm.

Elaine, Age 29, Dublin

Elaine received very little consistent advice or support to breast-feed in the hospital. She wanted to breastfeed and it seemed to go well in the hospital. Unfortunately, once she got home, it all went wrong. He was very hungry, she was in agony with bleeding nipples and she dreaded feeding him. 'After the second week I was so unhappy, I thought, "I can't do this", so I expressed and gave him formula. I don't really have an issue that I didn't breastfeed; I have an issue with the fact that I felt guilty that I didn't breastfeed, because there was so much pressure from the public health nurse.' She has subsequently met mothers who had very positive experiences of breastfeeding and are quite anti-bottle-feeding. 'They don't seem to understand what you go through if you can't breast-feed. That's what I find difficult, because they can be a little bit self-righteous about it.' She doesn't think that bottle-feeding has done her baby any harm. She knows she was a better mother because she was happier and more relaxed. 'I think it was the right thing for me, and I don't think I'll breastfeed any more of my children other than the first few days in hospital . . . I'll do labour, but I won't do breastfeeding!'

Alison, Age 38, Kildare/San Francisco

Because Alison was on very strong medication for Crohn's disease, she decided, after lengthy discussions with her obstetrician, that she wouldn't breastfeed either of her babies. There was no research to say that it was safe to breastfeed while taking the drug she was on. When her first baby was born the nurse wanted to fetch the lactation consultant to get her started on breastfeeding. It was on her chart that she wasn't going to breastfeed and her obstetrician had warned her she might get a negative reaction from the staff at the hospital. She asked for formula – 'You should have seen the look on her face: she was horrified that I would even consider formula.' The nurse brought the lactation consultant anyway. When Alison explained her decision, the consultant didn't accept it, and tried to persuade her that although there was no proof that it was safe, there was nothing to say it was dangerous. Alison was feeling very emotional at the time and the consultant continued to tell her that she was depriving her daughter of the best start in life. Thankfully her husband was there to back her up and help her stand her ground.

Yvonne, Age 40, Dublin

'I didn't breastfeed. It wasn't for me, wasn't my choice.' At twenty-one years old, she was very young and was very sure she didn't want it. After her third child, she did regret not trying to breast-feed him. 'Why didn't I just do it, even for one day, just to feel that feeling . . . It is one thing I regret.'

Tracey, Age 38, Westmeath

Tracey struggled with breastfeeding her first baby. She was extremely anxious about feeding, worrying that the baby wasn't getting enough food. She feels that this anxiety was triggered partly by her shock and anger at how badly the birth went. 'I just wasn't sleeping or relaxing. I couldn't switch off, was listening out the whole time . . . I felt very alone at night in the hospital, ringing the bell for help with feeding and latching on and not getting it because they were so busy and short-staffed.' She kept going, and looking back, realised the baby was actually feeding and latching, but she worried that she wasn't doing it right and was very hard on herself. After a very difficult first week emotionally and physically, Tracey was convinced she wasn't feeding correctly. 'There was a really good public health nurse that came out to me and she showed me how to feed my daughter lying down. I can remember having this one feed lying down where I felt that relaxing feeling that you are supposed to get after you breastfeed, and it was the first time I had relaxed in a whole week.' Having fed her for eight days she switched to bottles. Being so tired, she found this stressful too – having to figure out sterilising, teats and formula.

Emma, Age 33, Dublin

Emma breastfed her first baby for a few days in hospital. 'There was a point in hospital where I said "I'm exhausted . . . I don't think this is going to be worth the grief. I'm so tired." When I gave him a bottle, I just felt this relief, because he was a very hungry child. I thought that if you've big boobs, that's great, but it wasn't. It's a real hassle to breastfeed.' When her baby got colic a few weeks later, she felt guilty as she thought it might have been because she had given up breastfeeding. She has very little time for the breastfeeding purists on the online forums who just can't understand how any-one can give their baby a bottle.

Combination-Feeding

Kerry, Age 37, Dublin

Kerry's baby didn't latch on properly in the hospital. She combi-nation-fed her baby with breast milk and formula while they were in the hospital, to make sure he was adequately fed. It was a few weeks before he properly latched on. She laughs now when she thinks back to using the double breastfeeding pump at home in front of the television when visitors came, having lost all sense of pride or embarrassment. 'Had I known what I know now, I would have stuck with the initial breastfeeding and just felt a bit more comfortable with it, that I knew what I was doing. I'd persevere a bit more.' Her son ended up on both formula and breast milk.

Kerry felt guilty when she met other mothers who were still

breastfeeding, wondering whether she was a bad mother for not exclusively breastfeeding her baby. She wondered if she should not have been more prepared, read more books, done more research. 'Now, I'm thinking, it doesn't matter how much research you do . . . going with your gut is so much better. You are so terrified and can be so easily swayed by other people's opinions and then you feel guilty.'

Ella, Age 45, Dublin

Ella gave birth to twins a few years after having her first baby, who she breastfed. Her consultant was surprised when she talked about feeding the twins, but she really wanted to try, and was able to combine breastfeeding with bottles. 'It made things so much easier: I could breastfeed one and feed the other with a bottle.' She thinks that it was a life-saver because she didn't have to get up and prepare two bottles and listen to one cry while she fed the other.

Helena, Age 33, Dublin

Helena was determined that she would breastfeed, but she and her baby had their difficulties at the beginning. Her milk hadn't come in and the baby was hungry. She got conflicting advice from the midwives about what to do. One told her to keep her baby on the breast and the next one told her she shouldn't leave the baby to go hungry and should give her formula. After a few days her milk still hadn't come in fully and she ended up trying to combination-feed with formula and expressed milk. She was managing to get one bottle of expressed milk every day. 'After three months, I said, OK, I've had enough, I can't do it, I'm frustrated, I'm tired, I'm not happy . . . but I felt very guilty about taking away what breast milk she was getting.'

On her second, the same thing happened initially, although her milk came in by the third day because she kept her baby on the breast all the time. The midwife she had this time around gave her good advice that helped her milk come in. She thinks that she could have breastfed successfully on her first baby if she had got the right advice and support. 'I believe that any woman can feed her baby if she gets good advice . . . It's a commitment to get that milk to come and the first ten days is very hard, but if you're willing to make that commitment I think it's worth it.'

Little Gems of Advice

- If you're having a tough time feeding (bottle or breast), it might feel like it will never end, but you will look back and realise it was just one of many phases. This phase will pass. Nothing ever stays the same.

- Breastfeeding can be draining. Don't expect too much of yourself, especially in the early weeks.

- If, for whatever reason, you decide to formula-feed your baby, don't listen to the pressure from other mothers, public health nurses or midwives. It is your choice. Do not feel guilty. You have not failed your baby.

- If you can persevere, do. Breastfeeding is great when it goes well. If you decide to stop, don't be ashamed of your decision. You haven't failed as a mother because you aren't breastfeeding.

- No matter what research and reading you do before your baby comes along, reality can be very different. Go with your gut and do what is right for you.

- The few days after the birth in the hospital you can be quite vulnerable, so stick to your guns if you are persevering with breastfeeding. Be clear that you would like to keep trying, unless the doctors believe that your health or your baby's is at risk.

- If you're not comfortable breastfeeding in front of people, don't be afraid to ask them to give you some privacy. It takes a while to get used to it.

- Every mother and baby is different. Just because breastfeeding has worked for other mothers that you know doesn't mean it should work for you.

- Once your milk is established, don't criticise yourself if it's convenient to introduce some formula at a later stage.

- Many mothers received conflicting advice from the midwives at the hospital when trying to establish breastfeeding. The latch is very important: get as much help as you can, preferably from a lactation consultant, in order to get it right from the beginning.

- Consider attending a few different meetings in your area to see which group suits you best.

- Even though breastfeeding can be difficult in the beginning, many women find it is handier in the long run than sterilising bottles and making formula.

- If your attitude is 'try breastfeeding and see what happens', it's likely you'll fail at the first hurdle, because those early weeks can be very hard. You need to be determined and committed to it.

- If feeding your baby formula instead of breastfeeding means that your experience of early motherhood is a happier one, then don't think twice about it.

- If you're breastfeeding and having a bad feed, just tell yourself that you'll get through this feed, and see what happens at the next feed. Don't look too far ahead.

- Don't worry if you want to breastfeed and you have a small chest. On the basis of the interviews conducted for this book, small-chested women did not report having any more difficulties than larger-chested women.

- If you are nervous about breastfeeding in public, do your local research before the baby arrives. Identify the cafés with comfy sofas in quiet corners where you can feel more comfortable in those early days of feeding.

- Don't listen to the purists on the online forums who don't understand why women would formula-feed their babies: it's not poison you're feeding them.

Anne's Pointers

Breastfeeding is fabulous when it works well. It doesn't work for every woman with every baby. Sometimes it works for the first baby and not for the second. It doesn't, in any way, make a mother who doesn't breastfeed a lesser mum than the mother who does. There are lots of professionals there to help. There are also community schemes where a local mother will call to a new mother to help with breastfeeding. Don't be afraid to use some formula with a hungry baby while you and baby are getting to grips with breastfeeding, as it's harder to cope with a crying, hungry baby when trying to get the baby to latch on. Don't get stressed about it. Make sure you are relaxed and comfortable when trying to breast-feed: it will help both of you to have a more positive experience.

Notes

1. 'ESRI Breastfeeding in Ireland 2012: Consequences and Policy Responses and Explaining the Increase in Breastfeeding at Hospital Discharge in Ireland, 2004-2010', Dr Aoife Brick and Dr Anne Nolan.

2. 'ESRI Breastfeeding in Ireland 2012: Consequences and Policy Responses and Explaining the Increase in Breastfeeding at Hospital Discharge in Ireland, 2004-2010', Dr Aoife Brick and Dr Anne Nolan.

3. OECD 2009 www.oecd.org/els/social/family/database.

5.
Visitors

Visitors, while often well-meaning, can be a major source of stress when your baby arrives. Many of the women I interviewed regret allowing so many visitors in the early days and weeks. This chapter has some solid pieces of advice about how to manage them. A lot of first-time mothers fall into the trap of continuing to be a good hostess, making tea and coffee for their visitors and entertaining them, when they should be in bed. Everyone needs to have the chance to recover from childbirth and adapt to this new phase of family life.

Kate, Age 38, Dublin

There was always someone coming to stay at our house or people coming over for dinner. I am a sociable person, and I found that when my first baby was born, part of me wanted to see people and I didn't want to say no. I should have just put off the visitors for the first few weeks apart from short visits from immediate family. I wasn't able for all the visitors; I was too tired, but yet I really wanted the company. It's hard to get the balance right. On my second baby, I stayed in bed for two weeks, only getting dressed twice during that time. My in-laws came to visit after ten days and the only others who were allowed to visit in the meantime were people who came to help. I think I handled the whole 'visitors' thing better the second time round. I didn't let myself feel guilty about saying no.

Kerry, Age 37, Dublin

Kerry didn't sleep when her baby slept, because she would be putting on a wash or tidying up, partly because visitors would be coming and she wanted the place looking clean and tidy. She thinks new mothers are generally too polite. Why don't we let visitors make their own tea and why don't we just go upstairs to sleep when we're tired when visitors are here?

Elaine, Age 29, Dublin

Elaine looks back and wishes she had been more direct when visitors came. She would have liked people to wash their hands before holding the baby, but didn't ask. Her husband has a very big family and they had endless days of visitors in the weeks after they came home. She didn't feel comfortable with the visitors holding the baby. She knows that may have been a bit irrational but that's how it was for her at the start. 'To be honest, I didn't want to see anyone for the first couple of months. I felt revolting, I looked fat and misshapen, and I still had that deflated belly. I felt very self-conscious and I was still getting to know my baby.'

Jenny, Age 35, Dublin

Jenny and her husband lived in a small house with no guest room. This ended up being a blessing in disguise, as their families lived down the country or abroad, and no one could come to stay. After coming to visit during the day, they had to go home or stay nearby. 'It was nice to have that support structure for the first two weeks, but also that everyone went home at the end of the day.' They only invited their parents to come to the hospital the day after the birth. 'I just felt really protective and possessive over my baby. I felt like I needed to establish myself with her before anybody else came in and told me how to be her mother.'

Barbara, Age 32, Dublin

Barbara and her husband will never forget the ridiculous number of visitors they had. It was awful. She strongly advises that new mums 'limit the visitors . . . Only allow them to stay for a certain period of time. Do not make them tea or coffee. Do not encourage them to stay.' Her favourite visitor, an aunt, used to come for fifteen minutes and then leave. This was ideal. A friend of hers had an interesting approach: she sent a text to all of her friends and relations to inform them of the birth of her baby. A few days later she sent another text inviting them to the baby's christening a month later. She has a huge social circle and they have a very large family, so rather than having a regular trickle of visitors, they invited everyone to the christening. If Barbara was doing it again, she would allocate a particular day in the week for visitors. Alternatively, she might have all the workmates come together in one visit, or a certain gang of friends come together. She also thinks, if she had the energy, she would go to other people's houses instead, so she could decide when the visit was over.

Ruth, Age 36, Dublin

Ruth was happy that, on her first child, no one came to visit them, as she was staying with her mother-in-law. On her second child, people just popped in whenever it suited them, which didn't work well at all. 'People were just dropping up . . . when you're trying to get in to a routine, or you need a bath.' One visitor arrived with her boyfriend when she was breastfeeding and commented 'Oh my God, you're breastfeeding, I can't sit there when you're breastfeeding.' She knows now that she shouldn't have to put up with such comments: if they don't want to see it, then they shouldn't be there. With her third child, she wasn't afraid to put people off. She didn't allow anyone to visit in hospital except her husband and children. 'Enjoy the time in hospital . . . You need that time to recover.'

Cathy, Age 30, Dublin

Very few of Cathy's friends had babies and they didn't seem to realise when it was time to go. 'Overall, it was fairly positive. I liked having people coming and going. The worst visitor experience was when my partner's mum and sister came from the country: it was seven days after my daughter had been born and I still hadn't been for a poo.' While we were there, she remembers spending an hour and a half in the bathroom thinking, they really have to go soon! 'I was in so much physical discomfort at that stage and they are very proper. I just wanted to lie on the couch and whinge, and I couldn't!'

Laoise, Age 37, Dublin

Laoise stayed in her bedroom, which meant that people didn't stay so long and they generally made their own cups of tea. 'It was great. I had two chairs at the end of the bed, and people would come in and chat for a few minutes. It was lovely.' It was a lot more work for her partner, but she felt it was a great approach. Second time round she did the same, but improved it even further with DVD box sets and movies to watch.

Caroline, Age 35, Dublin

Caroline's parents-in-law lived in the UK. They came over to stay for two weeks on the birth of her first baby when he was three days old. Even though they were very helpful, she really didn't want them there so soon. 'We needed some time just ourselves, just to be on our own for a while, but they had flights already booked.' Her husband was downstairs with his parents and she felt really alone and overwhelmed upstairs in her room. On her second baby, she asked them not to book flights till the baby arrived, but they booked them anyway and arrived five days after he was born. After the birth of her first baby, she remembers coming downstairs to have meals with them, thinking 'This is not what I want.' After the birth of her second baby, she made the new baby her priority. Her in-laws were more helpful this time as they could entertain her older child. On her first baby, she had lots of friends who wanted to come around and see him when he was tiny. 'My friends have had their own children now and they can't believe that they rocked up to my house the day after we came back from hospital.' She now leaves it a few weeks before visiting anyone. 'I was conscious about breastfeeding in front of people. I had this big scarf that I used. You know how it is: boob out at the start, trying to get him to latch on. I was pretty much naked from the waist up.'

Sinead, Age 37, Cork

After the difficult birth of her first baby, Sinead and her husband asked people not to visit at the beginning as she really didn't feel like seeing anyone. After her second baby she was texting people asking them to come and see her, having had a very different experience. She says you just have to see how you feel when the time comes.

Alison, Age 38, Kildare/San Francisco

Alison was happy to have visitors at the hospital. However, things were overwhelming when she returned home; she felt she had to be getting up to make tea. In fact, all she wanted to do was sit on the bed in her pyjamas with the baby. When her first baby was a week old, her sister-in-law arrived at the house for a week with her teenage son. Alison asked for this not to happen when her next baby arrived, but to no avail. 'It's really difficult having people in your house twenty-four hours a day for a week.'

Megan, Age 40, Dublin

Megan is very sociable and knew she had to be careful with visitors.

'I scheduled visitors very carefully . . . I actually wasn't in a rush to see people. We only allowed one visitor a day and not for too long.' She advises getting people to come in groups, because then you don't have to do all the talking; they can chat to each other. 'I'd probably see even less people next time.'

Sarah, Age 37, Cork/London

Sarah was living abroad, so they weren't bombarded and were delighted to have some visitors to stay after two weeks. 'We had arranged with our families that they were never going to come instantly after the birth, but after two weeks they would come and stay.'

Gemma, Age 40, Dublin

Gemma's husband was appointed gatekeeper at their house with regards to visitors. 'As a first-time mum, you feel under a lot of pressure. Instead of being a little more relaxed about it, I was more sensitive about people staying too long.' She was in much better shape physically after her vaginal delivery on her second baby than she was after a caesarean on her first, and craved company. Her second son was born with Down syndrome and she 'was so keen for people to meet him as a baby' and see what a lovely tiny baby he was.

Ella, Age 45, Dublin

Ella enjoyed the large number of visitors they had. It had taken a long time for them to have children and they had a few losses along the way, so people were very happy for them and very positive towards them. Her husband found it difficult though, with all the teas and coffees that had to be made. It all depends on personality: she thinks some people need space, but she loved all the positivity and it was such a happy time.

Fionnuala, Age 40, Dublin

Fionnuala's in-laws arrived to the house the day the baby came home. 'They weren't offering to make tea . . . I was stupid enough to be making them tea.' She feels that she shouldn't have put other people ahead of herself, but then looking out for herself was never her strong point. 'I thank my son for that lesson; I think he's come along to teach me that.'

Suzy, Age 36, Dublin

There had been a death in her husband's family just before the birth of Suzy's baby. As a result, the whole family was around and everyone came to visit and sat in her room in the hospital for the day, including her brothers-in-law, her mother-in-law, her own mother, and her brother and sister-in-law and their children. Her best friends were there too. This continued when they got home, and visitors streamed through the door. 'Next time, I'm not leaving my bedroom; nobody's coming to visit. It's a week . . . You'll see him when you see him.'

Emma, Age 33, Dublin

There were far too many visitors at the hospital. 'There were people all over the place. Everyone was coming, all the brothers, all the time . . . and I was there trying to breastfeed my baby . . . I thought they'd never leave!' When she got home they continued to come around, 'and they kept bringing over chips, used my plates and didn't clean up after themselves!'

Patricia, Age 35, Dublin

Patricia's husband was very protective when visitors came to the house. He met them at the door with disinfectant and told the children not to touch the baby. They were careful to limit the number of visitors. 'I felt like there were lots of people who wanted to come, and they were there for when we were ready.' One of the nicest things that was done for her after the baby was born was the delivery of a bag of home-cooked meals to tide them over for a few days. She advises any new mum to get someone in to clean the house, allow people to help and not worry about how the house looks. 'Only let people visit who you don't mind seeing your house in a bit of a mess. Keep the other ones at bay for a while.'

Andrea, Age 38, Dublin

On her first baby, Andrea's parents came to visit at the hospital on day one. On the second day, her husband's parents had arrived rather unexpectedly, as well as her aunt and uncle. 'It was like they were in the pub . . . I found that really stressful. I was worried about how they were impacting on other people in the ward because they were really, really loud.' There were a lot of visitors at home too.

They were much stricter on their second baby. Also, 'people aren't that interested on your second baby.' On baby number one, she knows that she shouldn't have been entertaining visitors. 'I had to be this perfect housewife, mother and wife, and hostess.'

Isobel, Age 39, Dublin

Isobel and her husband invited a gang of friends over to the house four days after the baby was born, for a glass of wine. People arrived all through the afternoon and didn't go away: they just stayed on, drinking wine and eating crisps. She looks back at photos of that day and realises how crazy that was. She would advise any new mum to have either no visitors for up to a month, or ask people to come for ten minutes and then leave. The best visitors were those who stayed for a short time and brought practical gifts like home-made dinners and magazines.

Martha, Age 40, Wicklow

For the first two weeks, Martha had a lot of visitors, when in retrospect she feels she should have been sleeping. 'I felt very under pressure to still be the hostess when people arrived.' She was in a lot of pain after her section but found she was making tea and coffee when people visited. There were days when she just wanted to go to her room to feed her son in peace as she was having difficulty breastfeeding. 'I found it exhausting having people . . . It depended who it was.' People who were always easy to be with were a welcome distraction, but others were an effort. Due to a history of depression, she had been advised by a doctor to have no visitors in the first few days so that she would be able to sleep. Despite this, some people still visited.

Little Gems of Advice

- Let visitors make their own tea or coffee.
- The presence of visitors doesn't mean you should ignore your body if you're tired. Go to bed if you need to.
- If you are concerned that people are bringing germs into the house, don't be afraid to ask them to wash their hands before taking the baby.
- Limit how long your visitors stay.
- Consider having visitors come in groups, so they can talk to each other when you get too tired.
- If you have the energy, go to other people's houses instead of them coming to you: at least then you can control the length of the visit.
- Consider having the baby's christening/naming ceremony

while the baby is still quite young, and let everyone know that they can see the baby then.

- If you have a difficult birth, you may not feel like seeing anyone for a while. Don't be afraid to ask people not to visit for a week or two. Ask your partner to be the gate-keeper.

- Only have visitors who don't mind seeing you and your house in a bit of a state. Keep the other ones at bay for a while.

6.
Inside Your Head – Post Birth

My mind has never been as affected by anything as it was by the arrival of my first child. It was reassuring to speak to other mothers, and to realise that I was not alone, not by a long shot. There are women who sail through childbirth and early motherhood, or at least claim to, but I haven't met many.

Our mental health is precious and becoming a mum can take its toll, particularly in the first few months. The stories that follow show just how much the challenges of early motherhood can test our mental well-being.

Facts and statistics

According to the Center for Women's Mental Health (a joint programme between Massachusetts General Hospital and Harvard Medical School), about 50 to 85 percent of women experience 'baby blues' during the first few weeks after delivery. After childbirth, about 85 percent of women experience some type of mood disturbance. For most, the symptoms are mild and short-lived; however, 10 to 15 percent of women develop more significant symptoms of depression or anxiety.[1] Postpartum psychiatric illness is typically divided into three categories: (1) postpartum blues, (2) postpartum depression and (3) postpartum psychosis. It is useful to think of these disorders as existing along a continuum, where postpartum blues is the mildest and postpartum psychosis the most severe form of postpartum psychiatric illness.

If you are having a bad day or two, talk to another mother about it. Most mothers will have experienced the same thing at some stage, as the statistics above show. If you have symptoms of depression, you should speak to a health professional as soon as you can.

See the 'Resources and Useful Contacts' chapter at the end of the book for more information.

Kate, Age 38, Dublin

I hadn't found any mother-baby groups for mothers who were bottle-feeding. I went onto a mother-baby website and asked if there was anyone else locally in the same boat. There was such a great response that I had to close the thread when we got to eleven mothers (and their twelve babies); there wasn't enough room in our houses for a bigger group to meet. Those women saved my mental health and some of them have become really good friends. To meet every week and talk about things that to others seemed trivial, but to me were hugely important, was a godsend.

My baby was milk-protein intolerant, diagnosed only after six very tough weeks. We ended up trying three different types of formula and all sorts of other potential solutions to help the baby's digestion. In those early weeks, I woke up in the middle of the night (between feeds) and woke my poor husband to announce that I'd figured it out: the baby needed a slightly bigger teat to prevent her getting trapped wind. I was going to get up to cut a hole in the teat with a needle to make it half a size bigger. That would fix everything, I thought. I was off my rocker.

Things were psychologically easier after the arrival of my second child, as I knew that what I was feeling was mostly tiredness and that it would pass eventually, as it had with my first child. That being said, feeling exhausted still affected my ability to stay positive and enjoy my baby.

Sinead, Age 37, Cork

After a difficult caesarean birth, Sinead went home, and felt trapped and stuck in the house. She and her husband tried to go for a walk down the road. 'He screamed in the buggy; I was only five doors down the road . . . I had to turn around and go back. I was tired, I felt like I couldn't walk, and mentally as well I just couldn't do it . . . I think I had post-traumatic shock after the birth.'

When her first was born, she remembers thinking, 'Oh my God, this is my life, there's a tiny screaming baby, there are nappies all the time, I'm getting no sleep, I can't get out of the house, I don't know who I am any more. Oh my God, this is me.' She now knows that although that was the reality of her life for a short period of time, everything changes. When he got to three months things got easier, and again when he got to six months things got easier.

She doesn't know if it would have been possible for her to have taken this view if she'd received that advice. 'Even if things aren't how you thought they were going to be, it can still be OK; it isn't the end of the world. You're not in control any more. The minute that you get pregnant, you should probably realise that you are not the boss any more; it's out of your hands. You should make plans but you can't expect things to turn out that way.'

Sara, Age 39, Dublin

Sara and her partner had to go to a clinic when their baby was eight days old as there was potentially a problem with their baby's hip. 'I nearly had a nervous breakdown. I wasn't ready . . . I was terrified, a nervous wreck . . . I cried. I hadn't breastfed in public before and I was sitting there thinking what am I going to do if she starts crying; how will I comfort her?'

When her partner returned to work, she was terrified. The baby was just beginning to have colic. 'It's irrational really, but it's a real fear. I don't know what I was actually afraid of. I think I was afraid of him just not being there and whether I would be able to cope on my own. I used to sit there on the sofa for the first few days and tried to be all housewifey, and then the crying started and I realised I couldn't do that . . . so I sat there breastfeeding watching TV and watching the clock, waiting for my partner to come home.' Those colicky days she describes as dark, dark days, but they passed.

At one of their lowest points, when colic and reflux had taken hold, the baby was screaming constantly and they were getting very little sleep. 'We left her sitting on the bed, wailing her eyes out, while the two of us just stood there saying "What are we going to do?" I seriously said, "I'm going to call the public health nurse in the morning and see about adoption."' She knows she wasn't in her right mind, but at the time she was serious. 'I remember at one point, she just wouldn't stop crying and I shouted at her. I felt so guilty. This is something you couldn't tell anyone; you couldn't share that with anyone.' She remembers the relief when she finally told a friend, who said they had done it too. The inability to share this stress made her felt very isolated and alone. She wishes she hadn't judged herself so harshly at the time, and realised that she and her partner were just doing their best.

Martha, Age 40, Wicklow

Martha had a history of depression. She was watching out for postnatal depression after the birth of her son, and it reared its head after three months. 'I felt completely joyless. I had this lovely child and I just felt like I was going through the motions. I felt sad all the time and so tired. I felt very, very lost.' She found it hard that she wasn't getting on well with her partner. The day she realised there was something wrong, she was making dinner and her son was crying. 'I turned around and I screamed my head off at him.' Her partner heard her and they had a huge row over it. She was fairly sure at that stage that she had postnatal depression and went to see her GP. She didn't take medication, as she had had a negative experience with it before, but managed her symptoms through exercise and a better diet. It took quite a long time for it to improve. She felt that more support from her partner and reassurance that she was doing a good job would have helped a lot.

Looking back, she knows she should have stopped worrying about other people, about the floor being hoovered or about whether the meals were prepared. That time with her new baby passed very quickly and, as she said, she's never going to get it back.

Ruth, Age 36, Kildare

Ruth had moved into her mother-in-law's house for a couple of months as she was nervous about being home without help: she was only nineteen. 'My mother-in-law was a smoker, and I was so protective. In the evenings I wouldn't go downstairs with him and would just lie in the bed with him, feeding him upstairs.' She was amazed at how protective she felt. 'I remember the first bath on my own. You think you're going to let him fall and slip; you think you're going to break his arm . . . And changing his nappy, it's frightening, trying to get his hands into the babygros and vests.' The first time her partner left the house to go back to work, the baby was two days old. 'I was terrified, the day was going to be so long, he was working 2 PM till 10 PM. It was really long. I didn't leave the room; I wasn't happy; I just wanted him to come home.'

At the same time, Ruth remembers the feeling in their bedroom: 'Everything had changed. There was such a warm happy feeling. He changed everything: the smell, the sense around the place . . . You're just in awe, looking at them.'

Ruth wishes she could have relaxed more as a first-time mum. She remembers being very anxious, and hyper-vigilant about the baby being clean, and she spent a lot of time cleaning his belly-button and every crease in his body. 'You just need to relax and take a deep breath and enjoy it.'

Cathy, Age 30, Dublin

Cathy wasn't nervous leaving the house the first time on her own, or when her partner went to work. She does remember though how the day seemed to stretch out in front of her without her partner there. She found that the days turned into blurry messes. Sometimes, just a walk in the park changed her day completely and she didn't feel like the walls were closing in on her.

She loved all the new things that her daughter brought to her life. 'I remember looking at her in the first few days and thought, "I didn't know I'd like you so much!" You know when you meet people who have new babies and they talk about every little ridiculous detail? Now I know that it's fascinating.'

Mary, Age 32, Tipperary

Mary didn't leave the house alone with the baby until she was about six weeks old. 'I was terrified. I went for a walk. I was a nervous wreck. "What if she cries and I'm on my own, what if she needs a bottle all of a sudden?"' Her baby was a few months old before she brought her to the supermarket. 'I just couldn't hack it. I was nervous. She was fine, and she would have been fine if I'd brought her at two weeks, I know that now.' She wishes she had trusted her instinct more. Sometimes when people questioned what she was doing with the baby, it really threw her off. She knows that they meant well but she was so nervous that her confidence was badly affected. Her cousin advised her that as the mother, she knew her baby best, and she now knows that it's true.

Mary took an omega-3 supplement and flax oil to help prevent depression after the baby arrived: 'I really feel that kept my head above water. I didn't even get that low in the few days after . . . I know what it's like to have a low day but I didn't have much of that at all.' Her cousin also told her always to remember that tomorrow is a new day, so she was never scared of feeling a bit low. She just accepted it, went with it, and knew that the next day would probably be better.

Laoise, Age 37, Dublin

After the birth of her first son, Laoise remembers believing a lot of what was in the baby books. 'I definitely took all those books at face value. Other people who didn't seem as stressed as me had read the books and ditched them after a few weeks. I was mental with them. I was sure it was something I was doing wrong, and I really stressed out over it . . . I'd be stressing if he slept over three hours, when he was supposed to only sleep two, when I should have been kicking back and resting. If I could go back and talk to myself in those early weeks, I would say "You know your own baby best, and you can ring as many people as you like and you can check as many books as you like: chances are the gut inkling that you have about what the cause of the problem is, is probably right . . ." I've become a much more intuitive person, much better at reading body language, because I've learned to trust my intuition. As hard as it is, you kind of have to suck it and see.'

Caroline, Age 35, Dublin

Caroline put a lot of pressure on herself to get out for a walk when her first baby was only five days old. 'I didn't think that on my second. I knew he didn't need to get out: he was fine there with me.' People used to say 'You really should get out. Have you and your husband been out for a meal?' She doesn't agree with that at all:

they didn't want to be away from him, as they were happy being home together.

The first time she left the house on her own with her baby, she found it overwhelming trying to coordinate everything, including the feeds, changes, buggy and all the equipment. The second time round, she used a sling and it was so much easier.

'I remember thinking that I hoped we were good enough for him, I hoped we were doing a good job. I was thinking that he needs to have this particular toy giraffe. All the kids had it; I must find it immediately.' Again, she found that she didn't think like this at all on her second baby.

Caroline used to think that she needed to put him in a bassinet because he shouldn't fall asleep in her arms. 'People used to say things like, "Don't hold him too long, he'll get a feel for it." It really annoys me now when I hear it. Now I'd love if he'd just sit on my lap and cuddle into my neck, but he's too busy tearing around.'

Alison, Age 38, Kildare/San Francisco

Alison remembers coming home and feeling exhausted and very nervous. She was overwhelmed by the realisation that she was responsible for another human being. 'You're looking at this baby and you're thinking, this baby is completely dependent on me for nourishment and keeping them warm and safe.' She was an emotional wreck the first few days. 'You can read a hundred books about what's physically going to happen to you, but there's not a whole lot out there on the emotional side.'

The emotional surge she felt in the days after the birth was like the worst PMS of her life: she was crying for an entire day with no idea why. Life became all about feeds and sleeps. 'You think you're going to have a schedule, but you just need to go with what the baby needs . . . I thought I'd be all organised and have a schedule but that all went out the window within the first week of getting home.'

Astrid, Age 39, Germany/Dublin

Astrid initially raised her first baby in Germany, while her husband commuted to work in Dublin every week. Her daughter screamed every evening between 10 PM and midnight for a few weeks. She still doesn't know why. 'I found it very stressful not knowing what was wrong with her, and to have to bear this screaming every evening.' She did get some help from her family, but really there wasn't anything more she could have done.

The first time Astrid left the house with her baby, she just copied everything her sister did, as she had had a baby a few months beforehand. As a result, it didn't feel stressful. She does remember in the first few weeks, 'I didn't like people looking into the buggy. I was very protective: I nearly wanted to lean over the pram. I didn't want people to sneeze near her.'

She remembers trying to encourage her first baby to reach her developmental milestones, 'You can't wait for these things to happen.' She thinks that first time round, you don't know that your baby will just reach these milestones on their own. By the time the second one comes around, you just let them reach them at their own pace.

Elaine, Age 29, Dublin

Elaine found that she was hugely affected by hormones after the birth of her baby. 'The first few weeks were really bad. I didn't feel that I could talk to anyone about it. The thoughts I was having were horrendous.' She was paranoid that something might happen to the baby, and kept tormenting herself, imagining awful scenarios where she might drop her or hurt her. 'I'm usually a really positive person; I don't have bad thoughts.' The responsibility on her as the mother was certainly feeding this madness. 'The hormones really mess you up. I don't think anyone can understand unless they've been through it.' Elaine didn't have any friends who had babies until she started to meet up regularly with several other new mothers who she came across on an online parenting website. 'Suddenly I felt a bit more normal again. I thought, "Hey, this is great, we're all nuts!"' Sharing the day-to-day problems and worries of new motherhood made a huge difference.

Elaine often lost perspective in those early months. At eight weeks she started introducing textures to her baby. She was worried that maybe she should, at eight weeks, be focusing on her baby's development and started thinking that she needed to enunciate more clearly to help with the baby's speech. She can laugh at herself now, looking back, 'I think I went a little bit overboard because I was trying to be perfect.'

Jenny, Age 35, Dublin

'It might sound silly, but after the baby was born and my husband would come home from work, I thought, "She's probably really pleased to see you, because she's bored of me." You don't realise how big it is for them just to be breathing, and being in the world.' Now she looks back and thinks that it was ridiculous to think that she was bored in her company at just a few weeks old.

Jenny hadn't felt able to leave the house alone until two weeks after the birth. 'I don't know what I was scared of, but I just felt safer at home. Once I did it, it was like a little hurdle and felt really nice.' She remembers meeting a friend on that walk and asking her what kind of developmental play she should be doing with her daughter at just two weeks old. She realises now how ridiculous that was.

Megan, Age 40, Dublin

After the first three months of being home with her baby all day on her own, 'I thought that the monotony of the same thing every day was going to kill me. Change the nappies, get the breastfeeding done, visit a friend . . . That was when I had to do something and started baby boot-camp.' She would advise a new mother after those first few weeks, once you start to get back to yourself a bit, to plan two or three things a week to get you up and out of the house.

In the early weeks, 'I was so happy. I never felt so content after I had him; for once in my life I wasn't wanting. I should have relaxed a bit about getting out. It's only a short period of time.' In hindsight, she feels she shouldn't have been afraid of rocking and cuddling him too much. She was more strict than she should have been, wanting to ensure that he got used to sleeping in his cot.

She felt somewhat trapped as a new mum, seeing the space between feeds as her only bit of freedom. She knows that lots of women feel this way, but her personality meant that she needed the headspace. She remembers driving out of the house when her baby was eight weeks old, not knowing where she was going. 'I called up to a friend of mine and cried my eyes out because I felt so claustrophobic.'

Rebecca, Age 41, Kilkenny

After the birth of her first baby, Rebecca remembers intense feelings that came up in those early months. She remembers 'fear of something happening to the baby, fear of something happening to my partner, fear of not doing things properly or well enough . . . a bit of isolation too.' Walking in the park every day helped. She struggled with her changing identity after the baby arrived. 'I didn't know what I was any more. I didn't have my pay cheque. I didn't have any way of gauging if I was doing a good job.'

She tells any new mother that she meets that they're doing fine. Also, 'Enjoy it because it's going to go . . . Maybe the word "enjoy" is a bit strong but it's fleeting; they're going to grow up . . . Be open to those moments when they start gurgling, and all that stuff.' She knows that it's hard to appreciate those things when you're submerged in sleeplessness.

Sarah, Age 37, Cork/London

Sarah's return home after the birth of her first child was magical. It was a couple of days before Christmas and they had just moved in to their new house. 'She didn't leave our side for the first four or five weeks; it was really special.' She wasn't nervous leaving the house with the baby for the first time. 'I was so excited; everyone in the shops was looking at her. You do get very tired very quickly, but it was fine.' She loved the first few months at home, but does remember a few times when her daughter would scream for no reason. 'You just don't know what it is. It's not the usual colic pain and maybe happens for just one night. They're so small you really don't know them yet . . . That's kind of hard . . . You really are guessing.'

She felt fine when her husband left the house; he had to go back to work when the baby was five or six days old. 'But I remember him saying he'd get home between 3 and 4 PM . . . and he didn't. He said he had to stay later and I remember getting really upset and thinking that's really unfair.' Even now that the kids are older he hasn't forgotten how important it is for him to get home to them on time, as it's so hard being at home all day with the children.

Rachel, Age 41, Dublin

'I felt more vulnerable during my pregnancy than I ever remember feeling before in my life. I think it was the fact that I was solely responsible for the health and well-being of my baby while I was carrying her, even though I was supported by family and friends. It's a lonely experience in some ways and one we as mothers have to do alone.'

Rachel was blissfully happy in the first few months at home after the birth of her daughter. She never thought she would be able to have children. She was on a total high and this gave her lots of energy. it was much better than they could have imagined it would be. She had never been so happy.

She does remember though leaving the house with the baby in the car. 'Now I used to be a bit of a Michael Schumacher driver, and I think I slowed to about 26 km an hour in every zone.' She didn't have anxiety about leaving the house; her anxiety was when she left the house without her. 'I didn't want to be away from her . . . I felt physical pain being away from her.'

Yvonne, Age 40, Dublin

Yvonne was twenty-one years old when she had her first baby. The relationship with her baby's father was breaking down so she didn't want him to be that involved. She came back from hospital to her mother's house. Her baby wouldn't sleep and cried a lot, and she had no support during the night. She felt she came home too soon after her second child, many years later. Her sister had come to stay with her two kids to help, but actually that made the house very full and she found it stressful. 'My husband was self-employed and took two days off . . . I remember I used to stand at the sink and cry, thinking I was having a nervous breakdown.' When her daughter was six months old, Yvonne's mood was very low. Her husband didn't see how her mood was getting lower and lower, as he wasn't home a lot. 'I had awful thoughts; I thought I didn't want to live any more.' Her doctor told her she had postnatal depression and pre-scribed anti-depressants. 'I didn't want to be on them, but the doctor told me I had to because of the thoughts I was having.' She came off them after a year.

Looking back, she knows that she was upsetting her baby as she was exhausted and stressed. She feels she should have insisted that her husband come home at a certain time every night and she that this would have helped a lot.

Tracey, Age 38, Westmeath

As soon as her baby daughter was born, Tracey experienced severe anxiety and hyper-vigilance and was unable to switch off. 'About four days after the baby was born, I just ran away. I couldn't cope with these feelings . . . My partner knew I was stressed but I wasn't really saying it. I shut down verbally very quickly; I couldn't express what I was feeling.'

That morning she just needed to get away, to get some peace; she just wanted everything back to the way it was before. 'I hadn't slept for more than twenty minutes in five days . . . It was like being in a permanent state of panic attack.' What Tracey experienced was not diagnosed as postnatal depression, or baby blues. Her GP called it borderline puerperal psychosis (also called post-partum psychosis) but after further research she now believes it was post-traumatic stress resulting from a difficult birth experience compounded by a lack of sleep.

The feeding issue was a major cause of her anxiety, despite the fact that it was working, although it was hurting. 'I needed to let go of that but I couldn't. I probably would have helped myself if I had let go, and again, backed down on my plan . . . The mental anguish of feeling like a failure, and failing the baby.' She resented her baby for putting her through childbirth. At the time she felt: 'It was her fault that I had been put through the pain . . . How could she change my life like this. This was supposed to be good, but it was bad, it was all bad . . . I had so wanted her and now I didn't want her . . . I wanted my mum to take her or my friend to have her. I told them, "She would be far better off with you because I don't want her."'

Tracey knew deep down that her feelings were completely wrong. After three months, she eventually got an anti-anxiety drug and it helped her to be somewhat relaxed and looked at her baby a bit differently. However, when her baby was thirty weeks old, she started to have thoughts she knew she shouldn't be having and contacted the psychiatric ward in the local hospital, where she was immediately admitted. 'I was pleased that something was being done, and I was getting away from the horror that was my life at home . . . I knew it was time to get better.' She knew that if she could just sleep for days upon days, she would be fine and things would come into focus. 'I think it was a lot to do with my personality type.' She is a perfectionist and expected everything to be just right. She is very strong-willed and strong-minded and this, she thinks, contributed to it too. Six months after the birth of her daughter, after some counselling, she felt she was fully better. 'I had had no feelings; I was numb.' She started realising how crazy it was that she could have felt those things about her daughter: 'How could my mind have made me think she wasn't anything but the best girl in the world.'

Her second birth was a totally different experience. When she gave birth to her second daughter, it was straightforward and she had great support with breastfeeding. Even with all the pain and anguish of her first birth, Tracey looks at her daughters and knows that it was all worth it: 'You could never imagine how much joy they bring you.' She has just given birth to a third baby.

Kathleen, Age 38, Donegal

The first week after she came home, Kathleen couldn't stop crying. 'It was just that awful feeling of crying all the time. I wasn't particularly worried about not being able to look after this baby; I just wanted to feel better myself. It almost felt like a homesickness feeling, anxiety in my gut, not about anything in particular . . . that knot in your stomach that wouldn't go away.' She had a bit of baby blues with her second child, on day three and four, and expected it, whereas on her first baby it lasted a week. 'I just didn't feel as wretched. I was tired but just normal tired, not that crazy tired, where I had lost sight of the fact that I was tired and I didn't know what was wrong with me.'

Kathleen remembers being very anxious about taking their first flight when the baby was quite young. She planned the trip obsessively and packed everything. 'I remember thinking that this is almost an insurmountable task. How on earth are we going to get her on an aeroplane. I go now with two kids on my own. I could do it in my sleep.'

Michelle, Age 30, Dublin

Before she had her baby, Michelle didn't think her social life would change as much. At the time of interview, her baby was sixteen weeks old: 'I don't even think about my friends. Instead of a circle of ten friends, I think about maybe two of them, and generally they're the ones with babies.' She doesn't consider going out for dinner or a drink; often a coffee is as much as she can manage.

Anna, Age 37, Dublin

Even though on one level breastfeeding was great, Anna found that she often felt trapped. 'When she was hungry she would scream the house down, and wouldn't take a bottle.' Their first night out was to a show when her daughter was four months old, but they had to come home early, as she was screaming and wouldn't take the bottle of expressed milk.

Anna remembers being obsessed with the contents of her babies' nappies. 'Is she pooing enough? Is she peeing enough? . . . To the point of weighing the nappy to see how much wee was in it.'

Her firstborn had reflux. She remembers one night, about 1 AM, having a terrible time trying to settle the baby in the cot. She handed the baby to her husband 'in a completely psychotic mode, saying "Take that child away from me before I throw her out the window."'

Anna was also obsessed with developmental milestones. It was like a competition between the mums, whether it be about crawling, standing or walking. 'There's no need to compare or compete. Every baby is different; they will all hit milestones at different times.'

Gemma, Age 40, Dublin

Gemma thinks that women don't always support each other with their well-meaning advice, 'I have met some very arrogant mothers. It's very different for everybody. You hear people giving you advice that's black and white, [whereas] there's no middle ground.'

She remembers an overwhelming feeling of shock after the birth of her first son: 'Pregnancy was fine, but it took me a while to adjust to having the baby.' She is now besotted with her son. However, her experience with her first son was not the stereotypical one of 'love at first sight'. It was really only as she got to know her baby and had the closeness of being together that the intense love really developed. She appreciated the advice that she received, not to wish away every phase of his young life, waiting to move on to the next stage.

She found that having an excellent GP made a huge difference with regards to support in the early days. 'I would suggest that a new mother discuss with a close friend that they might need extra support . . . Put a little element of vulnerability out there . . . The loss of control is hard.'

Ella, Age 45, Dublin

Ella remembers well what she found hardest about those early weeks at home. She had been waiting for a long time for her first baby but she found the lack of control difficult. 'I was trying to be structured and organised and have a routine like I would have in my job . . . having control and structure . . . What I found most frustrating was that the baby just had his own routine and did his own thing, and it would change.' She remembers hanging up on her mum because she was rushing to the park as she wanted to be there by 10 AM. 'I felt that if I didn't get out early and stick to my routine, that I wasn't doing a very good job, that I wasn't in control.' Her mum advised her that she was going to drive herself mad, that the baby was only two weeks old, and that the baby was the one who should be dictating her routine. 'I thought I was back in work, but I wasn't.'

She knew that her obsessiveness about getting out and about wasn't healthy, but at the same time Ella wasn't the type of person who liked staying in bed late. 'I didn't find it calming or soothing; I need to be up early and dressed. Staying in bed makes me feel lazy and slovenly. But there has to be a balance between getting a new-born up and feeding and getting out, and staying in bed all day.'

She soon learned that not everything everyone tells you, and not everything you read, is a given. 'Every situation and every baby is different . . . If I'm asked for advice, my advice has been, just do what suits you, because everyone will give you different advice based on their experiences, their lives, their homes and their babies. If you read what you're supposed to be doing and you don't achieve that, it can be disappointing.'

Fionnuala, Age 40, Dublin

Six weeks after the birth of her son, Fionnuala had to attend a work event. She had been exclusively breastfeeding and became very anxious about how she would manage to feed the baby if he got hungry. She did not know where to turn for advice. She wished she had had someone at that point to help her figure out what she should do. 'This idea of support is back to the whole bigger picture. As a society we aren't that family-oriented; we don't have supportive communities around us. There are so many women presenting with postnatal depression . . . The emotional support affects every single part of how you parent.'

Fionnuala feels that so much of learning to be a mother is about learning to respect your baby as another human being. She feels that instead of trying to force him to do something, she should have just chilled out a bit. When the baby was six months old, she realised that the experience she was having of motherhood was valid in itself. It didn't have to conform to pre-conceived ideas she may have had. 'The baby woke up in the middle of the night . . . I was getting angry with him because I had to get up . . . I listened in the darkness and I could hear the song "Love Lifts Us Up Where We Belong" and I got a whole rush through my body and I suddenly got it . . . It was like somebody was showing me that I needed to pay attention.' It was almost like a spiritual experience.

Suzy, Age 36, Dublin

Suzy had major anxiety from about two weeks after the birth, and it stayed with her for quite a long time. Breastfeeding wasn't going well and she wondered if she was getting postnatal depression. 'I am really good at my job, and I really like being good at stuff . . . so I have to be really good at something . . . I'm a very alpha female and these are all soft things. My mother said to me that on day three my motherly instinct would kick in and I said, "What are you talking about? I have business acumen, I don't have motherly instinct." I felt none at this stage.'

She didn't feel she had the skill to feel her way through this period and try to understand her son. The breastfeeding difficulties didn't help. She realised after taking a break from the breastfeeding in the third week that she had been in a really bad place mentally up to then. 'I remember looking at myself in the mirror, saying, "You're supposed to be happy, you're supposed to be happy."' She hadn't told her husband how bad she was, but 'when you're in it, you don't know you're in it. What you're doing doesn't seem to contrast against the norm enough for you to feel able to ask for help.'

The anxiety that was embedded in her at that early stage still hadn't fully gone when Suzy did this interview, by which stage her son was seven months old. 'I couldn't be on my own too long. I was worried about the day, and that only stopped at about four months. I needed to know exactly when he [her husband] was coming home.' She feels that the anxiety was partly because of the presence of a latent anxiety that she carried her whole life but managed very well until she became a parent. She realised she couldn't keep a lid on it any more.

She would advise a new mother: 'Stop sweating. You can't plan it all. It's not going to be perfect. You're striving for that 80 to 100 percent; it's ridiculous. It makes you manic and kind of unbearable to live with . . . You're going to turn into that neurotic mother.'

Roisín, Age 38, Dublin

Roisín realised years after having her children that she was sometimes emotionally up and down after their births. She remembers getting irrationally frustrated with her husband, who was obsessing a little about how many times the baby had wet or dirty nappies. He was getting annoyed because she hadn't written down the nappy information one day.

'I remember getting really, really frustrated.' Her mum thought she had baby blues, and gently managed her irrational reaction. 'I was suddenly aware. I was like, Oh my God, she thinks I'm being crazy, she thinks it's baby blues. Just by the way she said it, I knew that I was being irrational.'

Deirdre, Age 40, Dublin

Deirdre didn't have much support at home apart from her husband.

'My mum had forgotten anything to do with babies and only came down for an afternoon and left again, and that was it. I was completely on my own . . . In some ways that's nice, as you're making your own decisions, but it's a big undertaking.' She feels that she was really winging it for the first six weeks.

She thinks that as a new mother, you feel that everything has to be done right, whether that means having the right equipment, or the parents ensuring that the family home is free of marital strife. 'There's this feeling that if everything's not perfect, I'm letting them down . . . when really if somebody changes their nappy and feeds them and they get love, that's actually all they need.'

If she could go back to her younger self as a new mum, she would like to reassure herself that she was going to be great at this. She would say, 'Don't beat yourself up about things. Do what feels right for you. Don't do things to please other people. Everybody's experience is different. Nobody's birth is the same. The birth that you will have will be fine, and you will get through it, and those first few weeks.'

Heather, Age 39, Dublin

One of the best pieces of advice Heather got was from her mother-in-law. 'She said, "Just remember it will get easier", and actually that became a mantra, particularly when it was really, really hard . . . She was right . . . It passes, and you forget the pain and the sleepless nights . . . and then you do it again!'

People told her that she would know what was wrong when her son was crying. She found that that wasn't true: she didn't know. 'You're going through it like you're blindfolded at first because you have no idea.'

In retrospect she knows she was right to trust her gut feeling, as there were problems with breastfeeding that turned out to be a breast abscess in her case, and a posterior tongue-tie in the case of the baby. She wishes she had got help earlier. 'If you feel there is something wrong, just keep persevering.'

Patricia, Age 35, Dublin

In the early months of pregnancy, Patricia was struck by the sense that she was fully responsible for him. 'You're jumping a generation in an instant . . . No matter how excited you've been about it, and no matter how much you thought you've prepared for it, you haven't got the enormity of that until you've got the baby. You don't just get it for a few hours; that was hard for me to get my head around. There's no going back, and you are fully responsible for another human being.' She found that it was hard to accept that you can't walk away from this baby without major consequences.

She got some great advice from a friend, who said, 'You have to just accept that for a six-or-eight-week period, you are theirs, and that's it. Just put yourself in that bubble for six to eight weeks. You're OK with it then, as it's a finite time.' In the early weeks, as she changed the sixth or seventh nappy of the day, she remembers thinking that she was going to be changing nappies forever. That thought felt very true for her at that moment in time (even though logically she knew it wasn't). At nine weeks she had her in-laws over to stay for a weekend; she cooked and baked and went out for lunch. She never would have believed in the early weeks that she would have been able to do that. 'I don't think you're ever going to be as vulnerable in your life as you are after your first child. It's such a seismic shift.'

She believes she had postnatal anxiety or some kind of post-traumatic stress. She was afraid she was going to mess up. 'I felt like I was the only person in the world who was going to be responsible for making or breaking him.' When people would visit and ask about the baby, she was able to tell them honestly that she was thrilled with her baby, adored him and was blown away by how gorgeous he was. But when they asked how the birth was, 'I would spend longer telling them about how awful my birth was and I'd be crying about it, and the baby was like a separate thing completely . . . I couldn't get beyond it.' Some people wouldn't allow her to talk about it and would tell her to get on with it, when she felt she needed to process it by talking about it in order to get over it.

Patricia always used the mantra 'this too shall pass' throughout her life to get her through difficult periods. It didn't work for her after the birth of her first baby. 'I expected to be so blown away with love for my child that I wouldn't mind getting up in the night; I wouldn't mind all the pooey nappies; I wouldn't mind any of it. But that's not really true. Maybe it is for some people, but for the vast majority of women, that's not true.' She then wondered if there was something wrong with her, or with her love for him, but believes that that's something that comes with time.

Her advice to a new mum would be: 'Don't fret. The intensity of this will let up in just a few weeks. I know this seems like the longest time of your life in some ways . . . but you're in the eye of the storm in those early weeks. Put your head down and get through it. It's a hard grind. Don't over-think it. While you mightn't get things 100 percent right all of the time, that doesn't matter.'

Julianne, Age 39, Dublin

Julianne was very weepy in her first week after her first baby was born. Anyone who came to the house saw her in floods of tears. She didn't have many people around her, as she lived away from her family, and that was difficult. 'I always said to myself, tomorrow will be better. I met so many people who said that this time passes so fast, enjoy it; and I still do it. I stop . . . and when I'm lying in my bed at eighty-something in a heap, I'll remember this day.'

After her first baby was born, they brought him to a cranial osteopath and to a paediatrician as they thought he might have had reflux. 'Actually what I think he really had was exhaustion. We didn't know it and we didn't read his signs early enough . . . He just wanted to be left alone to go to sleep. We were just naive and poking at him an awful lot.' She feels she could have been calmer and more relaxed and wishes she had just trusted that he would eventually go to sleep.

Andrea, Age 38, Dublin

In those early months of motherhood, Andrea was struck by how much she loved her children. She wasn't always sure if she wanted children. 'I had always assumed that the person I loved most in the whole wide world was my husband, and that my kids would come next; we were the unit.' However, she was amazed by the intensity of the love she felt when her first and second babies arrived. It was different to anything she had ever experienced.

Isobel, Age 39, Dublin

Isobel and her husband spent the first two weeks of their new baby's life trying to continue on in their old life as much as they could. They would get up and go out for lunch and a glass of wine because for the first time in their lives they weren't working and thought it was like a holiday that they needed to make the most of. 'In retrospect, I wish I had spent the first thirty days at home, sending other people out to get stuff.' After the first few weeks, when her husband had gone back to work and her parents had gone home, there was a period where she felt very alone and wouldn't see anyone for the whole day.

In the weeks after the birth, 'I was a basket-case; if you had asked me to pass the salt, I probably would have started crying.' She handled it really badly and developed some irrational behaviours because of excessively protective feelings towards her baby. 'I got my husband to fire the housekeeper because I thought she was going to steal the baby.'

Isobel found that things like baby equipment caused quite a lot of stress. They spent much of the early weeks sorting out a flood of new products and baby gifts. 'My first few weeks I just remember not having time to enjoy her.'

She thinks that men need to remember that their partner might be in a highly fragile emotional state after childbirth. She was in a very anxious state. 'You have to treat that with such tolerance and sensitivity. When the public health nurse called, I was actually paranoid she was going to take the baby away from me because I wasn't fully dressed.' Her husband exacerbated things by making fun of her mental state, but she feels, 'You have to walk on eggshells around the woman. Her body is totally altered; she has pain in her bum, in her boobs, and is feeling so unattractive. You have a sense of euphoria in many ways, but that goes very quickly, and then you're very much alone.' Isobel met a group of other new mothers shortly after her first baby was born and feels that this it saved her. She had days when she couldn't get a shower or get dressed, couldn't tidy the house with the baby crying all day. These days felt like her lowest days.

She wishes she had known in those early months that she was doing a brilliant job and that it doesn't last forever. 'Look at me now, it's 9 PM and I have no little baby to cuddle. On my second baby, when he woke during the night, I said to myself, "Do you know what, little buddy, I am going to enjoy you and I'm going to listen to your beautiful soft little breath, and we're going to enjoy this time together." '

Marie, Age 49, Dublin

Even though it was a long time ago, Marie can still remember crying when her husband left for work after six weeks at home with their first born. 'It was a sense of missing that support that had been built into us. Now it was gone, and it was my responsibility to fill the day. I remember being quite lonely actually; I didn't have a big support group.'

On her first child she remembers not knowing what was wrong with the baby and how frustrating that was. It was a bit easier with her second daughter. 'It took me time to get used to learning what she was trying to say with her cries . . . I wish I'd sat with them and watched them a little bit more . . . almost like a tracker, following an animal.' She wishes she had got rid of all the 'shoulds' in her thoughts around her first baby, like 'she should like having a bath' or 'she should sleep longer.'

Helena, Age 33, Dublin

When her husband first went back to work, Helena was very worried about him leaving her on her own with the baby. Day by day it got better and better. When their baby was three weeks old her husband asked if he could go out for a few drinks to celebrate the birth of the baby, and she was fine with it. 'As soon as he left I said to myself, "I can't do it. She is crying and I don't know what to do to calm her down. I'm not a good mother; I can't look after my own baby." ' She remembers that her mother-in-law came to the house at 10 AM one morning in the early weeks. Helena was having a bad day, and hadn't showered or dressed; the baby was crying and Helena was shaking. Her mother-in-law said, 'There is nothing wrong with the baby, she is just crying. You have to look after yourself. It's normal for them to cry; she's burped, fed and changed. Take your time, have your shower, have your breakfast. If you're not eating well, the baby is not eating well.' It made sense to Helena: if she was not well, she wouldn't be able to look after the baby properly.

She does remember being absolutely terrified to be on her own with the baby, and she couldn't relax. She had no experience with babies. 'I was really stressed and tense.' She had to learn that babies are actually quite strong and resilient and not as fragile as she had first thought. She had been afraid initially lifting her and getting her dressed. 'Definitely the first few weeks are the most difficult.'

Little Gems of Advice

- Look after yourself as much as you can. If you're not well, you can't care for your baby.

- If you're having a moment at home when you're drowning in routines and nappies, thinking that this is how your life is going to be forever, then stop for a moment. Remember that everything changes. All these phases will pass.

- If you think you are very anxious, try to find ways to relax and enjoy being with your baby.

- Try to take people's advice with a pinch of salt. Sometimes people question what you're doing, and this can be off-putting. You know your baby better than anyone. If there's any way you can follow your gut instinct, then do.

- Don't put yourself under pressure to go out of the house if you don't feel like it. Go out when you're ready, no matter what your relations or friends tell you.

- Don't listen to people who tell you that you'll spoil your baby by holding him or her too much.

- Don't be surprised if you feel like an emotional wreck when you get home from the hospital; you, your body and your baby have been through a major life-changing event.

- Try not to become obsessed with developmental milestones that you think your baby should be reaching. Every baby is different, and your baby will reach that milestone when he or she is ready.

- Hormones can have a huge effect on your behaviour and perspective. This, along with the huge sense of responsibility that comes with motherhood, can be really unsettling. Try to meet up with other new mothers as early as you can; it will help you to feel more normal.

- Once you start to get back to yourself a little, after the first few weeks of being at home with your baby, start to plan a few things every week to get you up and out of the house if you're ready for it.

- In the early weeks, your partner may not always understand how important it is that they come home when they say they will be home. Be very clear about why it is important to you, and that you need to know if they're going to be late.

- Remember that after having a baby you may experience a level of tiredness that you have never experienced before. You may think there is something else seriously wrong with you, but you might just be tired!

- The arrival of your first baby results in a loss of control over your day-to-day life that may be difficult for you to deal with. Before the baby arrives, talk to close friends about how you might need their support after the birth.

- In the beginning, don't try to plan the day with your baby as you did your work-days. We are used to setting goals and achieving them and it can be difficult to give that up. Mothers don't always recognise that caring for a baby all day is an achievement in itself.

- Every baby is different. If you read about what you are supposed to be achieving, and then you don't achieve it, that can be very disappointing. Do what works for and suits you, not what others say you should do.

- Learning to be a mother is about learning to respect your baby as another human being. Take the time to relax and observe him or her.

- Don't think that because everything isn't perfect, you're letting down your baby. If someone is loving a baby, feeding them and changing their nappies, that's actually all they need.

- A mantra that may help is 'It will get easier.'

- If you have a strong feeling that there is something wrong with your baby, keep persevering with the GP/midwife/public health nurse. The worst thing that can happen is that there's nothing wrong. At least then, you can get reassurance.

- You have to just accept that for a six-or-eight-week period, you are fully focused on that baby and nothing else. It's a finite time, so just get through it.

- The initial intensity of becoming a mother will reduce after a few weeks. When you're in the thick of it, that seems like a horribly long time. Just put your head down and do it. You mightn't get everything right all the time, but that's OK.

- Sort out all the baby equipment (e.g. buggy, steriliser, car seat) before the baby arrives. Know how everything works; this will minimise your stress in the early weeks.

- When you hear the word 'should' entering your thoughts, be aware that these thoughts are probably unhelpful, e.g. I 'should' be happy; the baby 'should' be sleeping; I 'should' feel more love for the baby.

Anne's Pointers

Try not to listen to too much advice from too many people. Even in hospital, different midwives could give different advice. If possible, pick one person you trust who has experience with babies as your 'go to' person, and use them as your sounding board.

I have listened to many women in those early months, when tiredness and hormones makes them think and do strange things. One woman had, when I arrived, put pictures of the family all around the Moses basket, as she had read somewhere that babies only remember the last face they see before they go to sleep. She wanted her baby to recognise its family when it woke.

Another woman asked me whether her baby will know that she didn't push her out, as she had an elective caesarean section. She was worried that the baby would hold it against her when she was older. I have also been told by mothers that their new baby is bored, and they have asked what activities they should do with them.

Mothers that I meet often think they aren't doing a good job of caring for their baby, especially in the first two weeks of the baby arriving. When I take a crying baby from the mother, and it stops crying, they often burst into tears and say they aren't doing a good job. A new baby is daunting, and scary, and arrives with no instructions. The need to be the perfect mother from day one is huge. I tell them to relax, take each day as a new day – enjoy the baby, and that it's never going to be perfect. Enjoy the moments as they come and you will laugh at the moments that were not perfect a few months down the road, when you are no longer walking into walls with tiredness. I try to get them to talk about why exactly they feel they are not minding their babies. Normally once they say it out loud, the feeling disappears and the tears go, and things improve. Don't be afraid to talk and to cry. It helps.

Notes

1. www.womensmentalhealth.org/specialty-clinics/postpartum-psychiatric-disorders/

7.
Public Health Visitor

The HSE commits itself to ensuring that a public health nurse will visit you within forty-eight hours of discharge from hospital following the birth of your baby. They will continue to visit you during the pre-school period. During these visits they will provide advice and guidance in relation to food and diet, including breast-feeding, bottle-feeding and weaning, immunisations and safety. [1]

Unfortunately, over half of the women interviewed for this book did not feel that their public health nurse carried out this role effectively. In fact, as you will read below, many of them found the public health nurse unhelpful and felt that their visit was a negative instead of a positive experience. It seems that it is all down to the individual assigned to your area. There were some individual nurses who provided outstanding support, going out of their way to look after the new mothers in their care. Unfortunately, many of them did not. Whether that is because of poor training, under-resourcing or lack of clarity about their role, something needs to change to make this service more effective.

Kate, Age 38, Dublin

My public health nurse arrived at the house the day we returned from the hospital. She was a nice, well-meaning and friendly lady, but she was clearly ticking boxes instead of listening to what I really needed to know. When she asked my bleary-eyed husband if he'd started to think about child-proofing the house, we realised that we weren't going to be getting much relevant advice from this woman. I had hoped to meet other mothers locally through the public health nurse, but was told that there was no group at the time for non-breastfeeding mothers, but that one was being set up. Six months later, I got a call from her to say the group was starting the following week. Thank God we started our own group here or we would have been very isolated new mums.

Deborah, Age 37, Dublin

Deborah had a positive experience with her public health nurse. Her advice would be that if you don't get on with one nurse, ask to see a different one, as there is often more than one. Her public health nurse said that there was a baby clinic every week and that she should pop in if she was having any problems. She found out that lots of mums were going every week for a chat and some reassurance.

Kerry, Age 37, Dublin

Kerry didn't find her public health nurse to be particularly helpful. In fact, she gave her one of the worst pieces of advice that she had received from anyone. She advised her to strap the baby in to the bassinet with the seatbelt in the back of the car for a three-hour car journey to visit her in-laws. She said it was a better way to travel with the baby so he could lie flat on his back. This is not a safe way to transport your baby! 'Had I been completely naive, I probably would have done it!' She recommends taking everyone's advice with a pinch of salt.

Jenny, Age 35, Dublin

Jenny asked her public health nurse to help her to give the baby her first bath. The public health nurse seemed surprised to be asked but did it, and it really helped Jenny. Apart from advising her to get her two-week-old baby on the school register, she didn't provide much other support. Jenny found that the midwives on the midwife-led scheme who visited her were much more helpful. She also went to breastfeeding groups where the public health nurses regularly weighed the baby and answered questions.

Ruth, Age 36, Dublin

Ruth never felt supported by the public health nurse on any of her three births; in that she always felt judged by them. When she went to the public health nurse for help on her third baby as a last resort, as her baby wasn't sleeping, it took three weeks for the public health nurse to get back to her.

Astrid, Age 39, Germany/Dublin

Astrid found her public health nurse to be quite competent. She was lucky not to need too much help; breastfeeding was going smoothly and her stitches had healed well. 'I think it's good to have somebody coming in, just to tell you that things are going well, so it's not just that you think they are going well.'

Rachel, Age 41, Dublin

Rachel was visited once by a public health nurse and didn't find her to be helpful. She had a very positive experience of childbirth and those early weeks at home, so she was surprised by how many times the nurse asked her if she was experiencing postnatal-depression symptoms. At the time of the visit 'I did think that if I was depending on her I'd be a bit lost.'

Emma, Age 44, Kildare

Emma found her public health nurses were of no help at all to her on the births of any of her children. She needed support, and thinks they could have really helped her if they had visited regularly and answered some basic questions that she had about feeding or sleeping. But they didn't. She felt they were just ticking boxes.

Barbara, Age 32, Dublin

Barbara had two public health nurses visiting her after the birth of her twins. One of them was really practical, and helpful, and instilled confidence. However, the other nurse, who seemed to have very little experience of children, offered very little practical help and was of limited use. A few days after coming home from the hospital, this nurse referred them to the baby clinic as she said there was a mark on one of the boys' hands that looked like a burn mark. Neither of them could see the mark, but as she was the authority figure, they didn't trust their own instincts and did what she advised. The nurse at the baby clinic, asked them why they brought the baby all the way in to see them, as there was nothing there to see. As a result of this experience, Barbara would recommend that if you don't feel confident that the public health nurse is giving sound advice, trust your own instincts and check the advice with your GP if it's a medical issue, or another more experienced mother for a non-medical issue.

Yvonne, Age 40, Dublin

Yvonne didn't find her public health nurse helpful. 'They were an absolute disgrace. I went down with my son one day really upset and worried, as he was screaming a lot. In the end he had reflux. When I looked at her she was looking out the window at the car park and I just stood up and left, and never went back again.' She really thinks they could be a great support if they did their work well. 'I know they're stuck for resources and everything, but still.'

Kathleen, Age 38, Donegal

Kathleen's public health nurse was very nice. However, she didn't really help her at all, but then Kathleen didn't need much help. 'I was shown how to change a nappy. I think they could have been a bit more "You'll feel like crap, this is normal".' She knew that they were ticking the boxes: she told them how she was feeling, and this may have put them on some sort of red alert. 'I did ask them when the crying would stop. They asked me whether the baby was crying a lot, and I told her I'm not talking about the baby, I'm talking about me.' They advised her to have a glass of wine, which did actually help!

Michelle, Age 30, Dublin

Michelle's experience of public health nurses is that they didn't take any responsibility. It felt like every time she asked a question, she was told to go to her GP. 'They must have seen this stuff a hundred times, but they won't commit to anything . . . They'll barely advise you to give the child paracetamol without going to the GP.'

Gemma, Age 40, Dublin

Gemma had a very positive experience of the public health nurse, who was the same person on both her births. 'She was warm, encouraging, practical. We didn't feel rushed, there were no silly questions, and she followed through on things.' She went out of her way to spend time with them, particularly after the birth of their second baby, who had Down syndrome. She did extra research on their behalf, and put them in touch with other parents in the area who had children with Down syndrome.

Ella, Age 45, Dublin

Ella had one visit from her public health nurse after her first baby.

She said the visit was fine but she could have done with more visits. She had lots of questions about breastfeeding, as it wasn't going well. One visit just wasn't enough.

Fionnuala, Age 40, Dublin

She found her public health nurse to be quite good, though some of the advice she received from her she doesn't agree with now, in hindsight. The nurse had advised her not to bring her son into the bed to feed him, and it wasn't until he hit six months that she realised he was better coming into her bed. She would sit at the edge of the bed, and once he was asleep, 'I would put him back into the Moses basket, and there'd be a squeak. He'd be awake, and it was not because of the noise, it was because he wanted to be in with me. I could have actually had sleep at the start by having safe co-sleeping.'

Suzy, Age 36, Dublin

Suzy didn't find her public health nurse helpful. She believes that the service is important and knows people who use the public health nurse a lot. She believes it can depend on who you get and would like to have had a voice of reason that she could have trusted.

'Any time I asked a question, they were so nervous to commit on an answer. I asked if I should feed him more, or less. The nurse said "Whatever you feel," and I felt that I needed her to give me an answer.' Some people need empowering to make their own decision, but at that time Suzy needed some clear guidance and didn't get it.

Deirdre, Age 40, Dublin

Deirdre found that she was receiving conflicting advice from the medical professionals she came across, including the public health nurse and her GP's nurse. Her public health nurse gave her advice about her son's injections but the GP's nurse dismissed the advice and wondered who had been advising her. She wanted to say, 'Are there no medical guidelines that you all follow or are you all kind of winging it as well?'

She had good support from the public health nurse after one of her births, and none after the other. She believes that it all depends on who you get. 'I think a lot of it is that you don't know what to ask them.' Her public health nurse asked a lot and probed a lot, but she could see that she was going down the postnatal-depression route. 'They're still very regimented in following guidelines. It wasn't brilliant.'

Emma, Age 33, Dublin

Emma found the two public health nurses quite helpful. The first time round, she asked them to check if the house was OK for the baby and if the cot was OK for the baby, and worrying that the baby was too hot and too cold all at the same time. The nurses did reassure her, even though she knows her questions were a bit crazy.

Heather, Age 39, Dublin

Heather found her public health nurses very nice, and they tried to be helpful. After a week with a roaring crying baby, the first public health nurse said, 'He's a little minx, just let him cry.' When the other public health nurse came to visit a short time later, Heather talked to her about the pain she was experiencing while feeding. She ended up having a breast abscess. The public health nurse advised her 'maybe you should take a glass of wine . . . but I suppose if you were a bit depressed it wouldn't be good because then you mightn't know when to stop and you might drink the whole bottle, and that mightn't be such a good idea.' She ended up not knowing where to turn for help.

Patricia, Age 35, Dublin

Patricia found the public health nurse good, despite them only having short visits. The repeat visit was helpful, when her caesarean scar was checked again, as it had been infected. She did call them once or twice with some basic queries, though in fact found the midwives at the hospital a lot more helpful.

Julianne, Age 39, Tipperary

Julianne had the public health nurse visit after the births of both of her boys. 'She was very good and calm and relaxed, and came back as many times as I wanted. She was helpful. I knew that if I had a problem, I could call her.' Her public health nurse offered to come up to weigh the baby after her caesarean so that she didn't have to travel to the clinic.

Andrea, Age 38, Dublin

Andrea's public health nurse was really helpful, she was very practical and 'no nonsense', in a good way. 'I can be quite embarrassed about my personal health'; but the public health nurse gave her a physical exam with no hesitation and made her feel at ease. There was no prudishness about her, and she found that really helpful.

Isobel, Age 39, Dublin

In general, Isobel found her public health nurse useful. She introduced her to a new mum on the street, but also was helpful at the local weekly breastfeeding meeting, while not being pushy about breastfeeding.

Rebecca, Age 41, Kilkenny

Rebecca feels that the nurse who visited after her the birth of her first baby did more harm than good. 'She made me worry that he wasn't getting enough food when I was breastfeeding. The scale they use is for bottle-fed babies. She was worried about his weight.' She fed the baby constantly for a weekend to try to get his weight up. The nurse who came to visit after her second baby reassured Rebecca that both of her babies were a perfectly healthy weight, and using that scale for breastfed babies didn't make sense. This nurse had been a midwife previously and was very helpful. It all came down to the individual.

Marie, Age 49, Dublin

Marie didn't find her public health nurse to be useful. In fact, she found her unhelpful. 'It's more like she was pointing out anything she could find that was wrong, as opposed to celebrating what was right. Now maybe that's just when you're quite sensitive with a new baby. I think she said something about my daughter's eye being slightly turned in, and that could cause problems later on', even though there was no problem with her eye. She brought up things to make her worry, rather than things to reassure her.

Helena, Age 33, Dublin

Helena didn't get one useful piece of advice from her public health nurse. She waited all day for her to arrive, and she didn't arrive as promised. Then they told her to come to the clinic instead, even though the baby was very young. 'Maybe it was because I was not Irish . . . but then I was hearing the same ridiculous stories [from Irish mothers] . . . It's obviously just how she is, a little bit ignorant I think.' When she did finally arrive, she wanted to teach Helena how to swaddle the baby. Helena told her that her baby doesn't like being swaddled, so they had decided not to swaddle her any more. 'The public health nurse said, "What do you mean? She is just a baby." She continued to swaddle the baby, despite what Helena told her, and the baby screamed the place down.

Little Gems of Advice

- If you don't get on with your public health nurse, or if you don't find them helpful, ask to see another one. There is often more than one in your area. The quality of the service you receive is often down to the individual nurse you get.

- If you don't feel confident that the advice you are receiving from the nurse is sound advice, double-check it with your GP for a medical issue, or an experienced mother for a non-medical issue.

- Write down the questions you have for the nurse in advance of their visit: it will help you to get more out of the visit.

- Ask your nurse to help you with anything that you might be nervous about, e.g. your baby's first bath.

Notes

1. www.hse.ie/eng/services/list/1/LHO/CavanMonaghan/Public_Health_Nurse

8.
Your Relationship

Having a baby can put a huge strain on even the strongest relationship. However, some of the women I interviewed described a significant deepening of their relationship with their partner after the arrival of a baby, despite tiredness and increased bickering. It seems that any weaknesses that existed in relationships before babies come along become magnified and more difficult to ignore. One of the most common sources of irritation comes from the change in the dynamic in the home. Many of the mothers interviewed felt that they were left with a larger portion of the household and childcare duties when their partners went back to work. Communication and a willingness to try to understand where your partner is coming from are critical in getting through those early months.

In this chapter I have included some thoughts from a few of the fathers I interviewed. Also, I have listed the concerns that many people have about sex after childbirth – something that many new mothers find hard to talk about. From my interviews, I have concluded that there is no normal waiting period for couples before they have sex after childbirth. It depends on a number of things, including the couple's expectations; how often they had sex before the baby arrived; how important sex is in their relationship; and the woman's physical and mental health after childbirth. Some of the mothers interviewed slept with their partners ten days after childbirth, whereas many others waited eight or nine months, or more.

Kate, Age 38, Dublin

My husband and I were so excited about the arrival of our first baby. We used to sit in bed, before the baby was born, and talk about what it was going to be like to have a baby lying there between us while we read the Sunday papers. We were so naive. I think our daughter was two years old before we ever got to read the papers in bed again, at the same time, and only because she was watching cartoons on the iPad! We miss that time together when we used to while away the hours on a Saturday afternoon lounging around at home. It certainly changes your relationship, but you'd never go back to the way you were. The baby makes life worthwhile, honestly.

We were always very kind to each other before our babies arrived. When one of us felt a bit down, the other would step in and give some much-needed support. Initially we were so exhausted, we were just in survival mode. We couldn't look after each other any more; we had to focus on looking after the baby and getting sleep. I really missed the kindness, and worried that we would never be the same again. I remember feeling angry with my husband about how tired I was, counting how many hours sleep I had had in comparison to him. I often envied the pockets of freedom he had when he went to work, and felt bitter when he came home ten minutes later than he'd promised. Those first few weeks we were both so drained, I don't know how we didn't kill each other; we probably didn't have the energy. Eventually, life got back to a different kind of normal, and we found each other again. We really needed to work at it though once the first few months was over, and to remember who we were before this baby came.

Deborah, Age 37, Dublin

Having a baby has really affected Deborah's relationship with her husband. Their relationship of over ten years is very strong, and looking after each other was something that came naturally to them. She was really concerned however in the weeks after the baby was born, when they were both exhausted and hitting rock bottom. It caused friction and tension between them that they had never had before. She thinks that she is more insecure now about her relationship than she was before she got pregnant. She never worried about her husband leaving her if things didn't work out between them; she always knew she would be OK. 'As soon as I got pregnant, I thought, "I am now anchored by this child; we are anchored. We will always have this child and you can't just walk away." ' Her insecurity was twofold; firstly she felt less secure in his love for her but secondly, and for the first time ever, she didn't know how she would cope if he left. The dynamic has definitely changed in their relationship, but not just negatively. He now sees and has great respect for strengths in her that he never saw before.

Kerry, Age 37, Dublin

Kerry and her partner have a strong long-term relationship. 'The demon comes out with lack of sleep.' They were at each other's throats at certain points due to lack of sleep and tiredness. Despite agreeing to share duties, one of them would be more tired than the other. 'Childishness would come in to play . . . It's your turn, no it's your turn.' However, any bad feeling was very quickly rectified the next day. She feels it's important to acknowledge what was actually happening so that it doesn't spiral out of control. Kerry and her partner were always very independent within their relationship and all of a sudden they were spending all this time together in the house. 'Be prepared that it will change your relationship, and just keep a bit of perspective. It won't always be like this; things will settle down. Sleep deprivation can really alter the dynamic for a while.' She says that, long term, it hasn't affected them: they have a new bond because of their love for their baby.

Elaine, Age 29, Dublin

The arrival of a grandchild brought up major problems with Elaine's in-laws, and resulted in her having to give her husband an ultimatum to do something about his family's behaviour. It was very difficult for their relationship, but it did get sorted out in the end. Looking back, she wishes she had not projected such a confident image, and had asked her husband for more help. 'I didn't want him to worry. I wish I had involved him a bit more. I wish I had explained to him what was going on in my head in the early days, instead of trying to be so strong.'

Jenny, Age 35, Dublin

Jenny and her husband had decided that during the birth, he was going to stay up near her head, as neither of them had any wish for him to see the baby coming out. However, the way things happened, he ended up seeing the baby being born. 'He saw my body in a way that I didn't want him to see it. Until that point you are a sexual being, and his wife, and your bits are there for different things, and I didn't even know what he could see. That lingered after the birth a little.' Next time they'll try to be clearer in their communications to the midwives about it.

Jenny feels that when it comes to the physical and emotional aspects of her relationship, it took a lot longer than she thought it would for things to feel more normal. If you're breastfeeding, 'your body is on call all the time, and your boobs are filling up or spraying. You don't really see yourself as a sexual being.' She thinks new parents shouldn't expect too much from each other emotionally either. 'There's not very much left for yourself at the end of the day ... You're really tired ... It's too much to expect to be able to have midnight conversations about how wonderful things are.' She thinks that a breastfeeding mother may need space to focus on the baby. It doesn't mean she loves her partner any less, or that she doesn't want to be with them, but her body is going through something huge, and she has to be on call numerous times throughout the day and night to feed the baby.

Her husband was great – patient and understanding – but it was important to her to get back on track sexually. She felt that the absence of this in the first year had a wider effect on her relationship. Certainly for the first few months, she thinks a new mother should give herself plenty of time to come round to the changed relationship.

Martha, Age 40, Wicklow

Martha and her partner didn't live together full-time until the end of her pregnancy. She worried about how having her son would affect her relationship. The exhaustion took its toll and her partner did have to take a back seat for a while. 'I have loads of experience with babies, but I could always hand them back. It is very different when you have your own baby.' Martha found she was still trying to be 'Mrs Fantastic,' having lunches and dinners ready, and felt that the expectation was there on her partner's part also that she would continue to do all this work at home, despite the new baby and having had a caesarean section. 'I found that very difficult, and I had the added worry, which I put into my own head, of "Is this relationship going to make it?" '

Martha felt like a bit of a Stepford wife by the end of her maternity leave. Her world became minute and she started staying home instead of going out to meet friends, so that she could make meals for her husband and continue to be a homemaker. 'Where did that come from? I was never like that before.'

Sara, Age 39, Dublin

Sara and her partner argued like they had never argued before. 'We both have very strong opinions and we certainly would have been able to argue, but nothing at this level . . . That was really hard.' However, her partner slept in the spare room when their baby was born, as she was breastfeeding, so he was getting great sleep for the first few months. Because he was getting decent sleep, he was able to take the baby as soon as he got in from work, to give her a break. If she was doing it all over again, she would say to him that they need to 'try to recognise the fact that it's really difficult. We're both really, really tired, that I do love you, and that anything I say over the next three months I don't really mean.'

Cathy, Age 30, Dublin

Cathy thinks she became closer to her partner after their baby was born. He was very involved and is very practical. 'He was really good at making sure that we were OK . . . I really appreciate that about him now; I probably didn't appreciate that before. Having a baby is one of the most stressful things you will ever do in your entire life. You wouldn't want to be having a baby to fix anything [in your relationship].'

Mary, Age 32, Tipperary

Mary hadn't really thought about how having her baby would affect her relationship with her husband. 'It actually made it so much better. We are so much closer; I hadn't really thought of it and it was a really nice surprise . . . We would bicker anyway, so it wasn't anything out of the ordinary. It was just lovely, and the pregnancy brought us closer as well.' She was nervous about the first time they slept together after the birth, nervous about the scar opening, about pain, and if she would be all floppy inside, but it was fine. She was glad to have crossed that hurdle when they did.

Barbara, Age 32, Dublin

Looking back to the first few months after their twin babies were born, Barbara realised that she and her husband hadn't experienced this kind of stress on their relationship before. In previous times of stress, one of them was always in a position to offer support to the other. 'In this situation, you're both so affected by the presence of a new baby, and the lack of sleep, that neither of you are in much of a position to offer the other one support. You're not really acting like a couple; you're just acting like two individuals in a traumatic situation.' This improved once they both started getting more regular sleep and they got back to being kind and decent to each other again.

Laoise, Age 37, Dublin

In the few weeks after their first baby was born, Laoise and her husband were both up every night doing the feeds and nappy-changes. The sleep deprivation led to uncharacteristic bickering between them. 'I was at home full-time and he was going out to work. I remember one day getting mad at him for taking the skin off a banana and leaving it on the counter, and I said, "Do you think I'm the help around here?"' She also realised that she had to back off and let him care for the baby his way, like 'putting the babygro on backwards and the nappy half falling off; otherwise I'd end up doing everything.' She thinks that becoming a mother challenges relationships. You start thinking that because you're at home you should be doing all the chores, instead of leaving them as shared chores, as before. 'We had to have a few conversations about that, because it is a really big change in the relationship . . . I would become resentful if I did everything in the house. To agree a division of labour is a good idea. Minding the baby is a full-time job, I'm not at home staring at my navel.'

Caroline, Age 35, Dublin

Caroline and her husband were pretty tired, and for a while it felt like they were ships passing in the night, but they got through it fine. Her husband was a great cook, and really looked after her, bringing her food and snacks. Caroline feels that it makes all the difference when you have someone to look after you. The lack of sleep made them bicker a bit more than before, having that 'who's more tired than who' competition.

Sinead, Age 37, Cork

Sinead feels that having children changes everything about you, so it has to change the dynamic between you in some way. She thinks it has made them stronger, as they had a tough time on their first baby. They had to really pull together. They had two children under two, which led to five years of disturbed sleep. 'The thing that got us through it was making time for each other.' Whenever they had a few hours, they would try to do things they used to do before they had children, like watch TV comedy shows or have a take-away pizza and a glass of wine. She remembers thinking, 'I married someone who is one of my very, very good friends. I couldn't have done that with someone who wasn't a good friend. You have to have a bit of mutual respect, and you have to look after each other a little bit.'

Alison, Age 38, Kildare/San Francisco

Alison feels that having children has brought herself and her partner even closer. She attributes this to the nature of their relationship and the fact that they were together for such a long time; he knows her better than she knows herself. He took on a lot of the bottle-feeds, which helped her a lot.

Astrid, Age 39, Germany/Dublin

Astrid's husband was very shocked by the difficult birth of their first baby; it took him a long time to get over it. She was in

Germany for the first four months after the birth, and her husband was in Ireland. Luckily, she had family to help her, but says: 'It was hard that we lived different lives.' She found that when he was there with her at the weekends, he found it difficult to adjust to the slower pace of their lives. They would have been very active before, hiking and being outdoors at weekends. 'It was a bit difficult to find a good balance.'

Megan, Age 40, Dublin

Megan has found that her relationship is better since their son was born. 'I was worried that my partner wouldn't be as helpful as he was, and that he would complain about tiredness, but he surprised me, in a positive way.'

Rachel, Age 41, Dublin

'The night before I went in to hospital, I sat on the couch and cried, because I thought this was the end of us as a couple, and what if the baby isn't nice? What if we don't bond?' After the baby arrived, they were blissfully happy. Her partner was at home for all of her maternity leave. Having the baby definitely brought them closer.

Michelle, Age 30, Dublin

Having their baby girl was really good for their relationship at the beginning. As their baby's sleep became more disrupted after about four months, things became a bit more difficult. 'He is now going to work shattered, so he's cranky. I'm cranky because I don't feel like my day is considered proper work, even though I'm minding her all the time. Maybe it's woman's guilt, but I'm getting a bit annoyed by that.' When her husband says he's going up to the pub to meet a couple of mates, it irks her. On one level she doesn't mind, but on another level she feels that her independence has been more compromised than his. Her husband didn't seem to be prepared to choose between going to the gym or meeting friends for a drink. There was time to do both before the baby arrived; now she needed him at home more of the time.

Rebecca, Age 41, Kilkenny

Division of workload and comparing who was getting more sleep were the areas of contention in Rebecca's relationship with her partner. It also changed the dynamic a bit, as she struggled with her changing identity. 'He was out working and I was at home with the baby. I felt like I had less power. It's a big thing to go from earning a pay cheque to doing something that's so much harder but which you get nothing for.'

Anna, Age 37, Dublin

Anna remembers, after the birth of her second baby, 'bawling crying because I missed my husband; I missed the relationship I had with him; I missed the closeness. We're only reconnecting now.' Her second child is almost three years old.

With hindsight she would do things differently. Before they had children, they did everything together. 'From the point at which my daughter was born, we sort of drifted . . . Before the child was born if I had had to save either my husband or my unborn child out of a burning fire, I'd have picked him. Within three or four months of the birth, if someone had given me the same choice, I would have chosen my child. That got even stronger on my second.'

Anna used to think that the way she looked after her daughter was the right way. She got sound advice from an ante-natal teacher that just because the way *she* did something with her baby worked for her, didn't mean it would work for the father. He needed to be allowed to do things his way. In addition, if she was doing it again, she would have copied what her parents did. 'They went out together every Tuesday and every Friday. I should have tried harder to get a babysitter.'

Gemma, Age 40, Dublin

Gemma feels that her relationship with her husband took a hammering. 'I was irritable and very, very tired, and while he was trying his best to be supportive, I probably lashed out at times. When that's sustained over a period of time, it really takes its toll.' In the first few weeks, she remembers telling him she hated him, but now can't remember why. She thinks it's sensible to have a chat about it before the birth, or to get your partner to talk to their friends who have had kids about how it has affected their relationships.

Gemma knows that they made a number of fundamental mistakes in the approach to their relationship after the birth of their first baby. 'Everyone deals with things differently, and you should make up your own mind about what works for you and your partner. Make time for yourselves without the buggy, and make time for yourself.' She feels she still hasn't done that, two years on. 'Some women boast that they haven't been apart from their baby for more than an hour, ever.' She doesn't necessarily see this as a good thing, but as pressure to be the perfect mother.

Ella, Age 45, Dublin

Ella and her husband had been through many years of trying to have children. By the time her first baby came along, she felt that the hardest part was over. Admittedly, they didn't have as much time for each other, and the baby became the priority for both of them. 'There was less romance, less personal time and less intimacy, unless it involved lying on the bed with the baby.' They tried to sleep together after twelve weeks, but it didn't quite work. Her breasts started spurting milk and they decided that her body just had other priorities at the moment, so they waited another few months. 'I think once we were both OK with it, and we told each other we still loved each other, the physical side of things could wait.'

Fionnuala, Age 40, Dublin

Fionnuala felt that she and her husband were joined at the hip before their baby came. 'There is a separation between us: our roles became very clearly defined after a few weeks. It's definitely been a big stress for us.' Before her baby was born, she remembers getting upset thinking about losing what they had together as a couple. 'Then the baby came along, and a few days into it, I thought, "I don't want this any more. How did I end up in this?" Thankfully my husband was the voice of reason and said that it was the three of us now, not us two and him, but the three of us.'

Getting time together without the baby has been almost impossible. She wishes she had been kinder to her husband. She resented him for a long time because she was breastfeeding and so was the one who was always getting up at night. 'We have become more creative about how we get time to talk, but time to do anything else? . . . I don't know how we would have a second child!'

Suzy, Age 36, Dublin

Suzy's husband was amazing in the first couple of weeks. However, as she started to get her head around what they were doing, her husband was happy to let her take the lead. 'He could get the basic survival stuff, but any of the routine things, he just didn't want to get. It's just not his way.' She remembers him asking her what military schedule were they on that day. 'He felt that it was imposed by me, which it probably was, but for the goodness of him being able to get sleep.' He doesn't cope well without sleep.

After the first few weeks, they fought all the time. She felt that this wasn't too serious; they used to bicker anyway. She thought that they were just in the middle of this crazy time and they would be fine, and that all would be forgiven. 'But after a couple of weeks he told me, I can't do this, we can't live like this . . . and he was right.' They had to sort it out.

Deirdre, Age 40, Dublin

Deirdre and her husband never really argued until they had children. 'The big thing for us is, and still continues to be, the feeling that you have to be in it fifty-fifty. If I feel I'm giving 60 percent and he's giving 40 percent, that causes the biggest arguments on both sides.' She feels that if you can describe to your partner how you're feeling, and if you can be respectful of each other, it will help you through it. It can be hard for your partner to find their role in parenting, as the mother's role is often so much clearer.

Emma, Age 33, Dublin

Emma and her husband had a very active social life before she got pregnant. Having children definitely affected her relationship with her husband. 'My son was really attached to me, and I was the one doing the night-feeds most of the time.' 'When I got pregnant, that all had to stop for me, but life didn't really change that much for him. It is hard not to resent that.' It is challenging to balance the needs of one partner going back to work, and someone having to do the night-feeds.

Heather, Age 39, Dublin

Having their baby definitely added a huge strain to Heather's relationship with her husband. They were not married long, but she wonders if maybe that's a good thing because it's almost always been the three of them. 'Breastfeeding can be an issue in a relationship, because the man is really very excluded, so you have to find other ways to include them . . . That's the one thing they can't help you with.' Having the baby brought them closer in another way, but she feels that you really need to be prepared for this strain on the relationship when your baby arrives.

Heather now realises that her husband probably needed more breaks from parenting, even though he got to go to work while she stayed at home. He was very hands-on, but 'he needed to have an evening where he's not helping with the bottles . . . although not really at the beginning; I needed the support then.' She felt that without that break, men start to worry that it's going to be like this forever.

Patricia, age 35, Dublin

During a difficult part of a very long labour, Patricia was getting sick from contractions. Her husband looked at her, smiling sympathetically. 'I remember thinking, thank God I have him; I can trust him; he'll mind me. I knew I could depend on him.' It did deepen the love between them. 'Of course, over the next six or eight weeks, there were times that through tiredness and crankiness we were irritating each other and snapping . . . but it was real surface stuff. That really deep feeling was still there, and still is.'

Julianne, Age 39, Tipperary

Now that Julianne is home with her children, she and her partner do see each other more than they did before. 'We do scrap a bit more, but usually that's about getting our son to bed, because he wants to let him stay up.' Overall, she thinks having a baby has been good for their relationship.

Andrea, Age 38, Dublin

The first two weeks after the birth of their first baby was great, as Andrea's husband was off work and she really felt like they were a team. 'When he went back to work, it got really tough. He would head off and I mightn't hear from him during the day. We had agreed that he would try to get home by 6.30 PM to help with bedtime routine, and gradually that got pushed back and back, and then he wasn't getting home till 8 PM.' She found that she could do the whole day with the baby, as long as she knew he was going to be home at a reasonable hour. That hour from 5 to 6 PM can be a baby's witching hour, as it was for her baby: she just wouldn't settle. She would wait for him to come home at 6.30 PM and because he was late, she would be annoyed. 'Then the next time he would come home that bit later because he didn't want to come home.'

In retrospect she thinks that it's important that the partner is very involved from the beginning. She took a lot of the responsibility for everything that was baby-related. She knows her husband would say that he thought she could do everything much better than he could. 'That made him feel inadequate, so it made him feel more like just leaving it to me, and I felt that he was dumping it on me.' Instead of talking about it, the resentment built up between them. She didn't understand why she had to explain it to him. She felt that he should just have known how to behave.

Having children, she believes, definitely changes your relationship. There's a strain that's put on that relationship. 'We have had to work very, very hard on our relationship. We're doing quite well. I'm not sure whether there were things in our relationship that we didn't need to deal with before we had kids. Having kids meant we had to deal with things that otherwise we could have just ignored.'

Isobel, Age 39, Dublin

Having children has had an awful effect on Isobel's relationship with her husband. 'I think I'm better when I'm working. When I went back to work after having my first baby, then our relationship got back on an even track.' She feels that her husband didn't understand what she was going through at home. 'I was quite deranged after having my first baby, with the tiredness, the newness of it all, the sense of responsibility. I hankered after my old life.'

She experienced major resentment building up towards her husband due to the unequal division of labour at home. 'I think he actually took advantage of the fact that I was at home in order to do less than he had ever done around the house.' When she challenged him about this, his answer was that he would employ a cleaner. Isobel didn't want to have a stranger in the house; she wanted her husband to be more involved. She knows it's partly her fault, as she would have pampered him in the early days, before they had children. 'I thought having a child would bring us closer together, but it's really pushed us apart . . . It's probably just widened the cracks that were tiny little fissures and were things I could skim over and accept.' Looking back, she thinks she should have made 'couple time', got a babysitter and made use of family members who offered to mind the baby so that they could go out. 'You have to nurture your relationship.'

With regards to the fundamental changes in their relationship, 'I allowed that to happen. It's my fault as much as his . . . I definitely allowed the relationship to die . . . He would say we're brilliant co-parents but we're no longer what a husband and wife should be, and he's right. I shouldn't have allowed that to happen, and hopefully it'll come back again.'

Marie, Age 49, Dublin

Marie's relationship with her husband did change, in so far as they went from a two-person to a three-person group. 'My focus, particularly in those first six months, was totally on the baby. Our times of being together were times of celebrating having her, or focusing on her, or nurturing her. She really became the centre . . . The focus went off us and on to her.' She felt that although having a baby changed their relationship, it wasn't a bad thing. Her husband was OK with that and he continued to look after her, even though her focus was more on the baby. He understood that her job as the primary carer was of great importance, and it didn't damage their relationship at all.

With regards to sex after childbirth, Marie advises any couple having a new baby to discuss this before the baby comes and to make sure that you understand each other's expectations and keep the lines of communication open. 'If it's important to you and you want to do it, then do it.'

The Dad's Point of View

Paul, Age 36, Dublin

When their first baby was born, Paul thought that his wife felt very resentful of the amount of time he spent at work. 'In retrospect, I didn't appreciate that she was getting really pissed off with me. It was a mixture of her not telling me and me not seeing the signs. I think maybe a lot of men do this, but I didn't think, "What does she need?" I wasn't particularly connected to her. For a while we were two separate people looking after a little baby.' He feels this was down to poor communication as well as anxiety, his inclination being to retreat into a little bubble in times of stress. He believes 'if there are stress fractures in a relationship, a baby will turn them into breaks. If things aren't going particularly well beforehand, this exposes them.'

He thinks that new mothers need to say supportive things like: 'You're being a great dad; I need you to be a better husband at the moment.' He believes that most dads are trying their best, as are the mums. Sometimes we need to be more honest with each other and communicate our needs. His wife would give the impression of being in control and on top of things, and he probably needed to be told that he was needed. 'There's a lot of pride and pressure involved in being a new mum. If you can't say to your husband "I need you", then it's very hard to say it to somebody else. He knows now that in those early months he should have told his wife more often what a fantastic mum she was. He wishes he had told her that she was amazing, and doing a brilliant job. This may have helped her to feel more respected and valued.

Paul sees it as a bit unfair on any new dad to have their screaming baby thrust at them when they walk in the door. 'A dad at work, is still at work. That itself can be tiring and stressful,' especially if the work is high-pressure and demanding. Often, he had said he would be home at 6 PM. He would arrive home at 6.10 PM and his wife would be furious. He didn't understand why she got so annoyed with him. It took him a long time to realise that when she was there in the house with the kids on her own, 6 PM was the time when the cavalry was coming to her rescue, when the prison door opened. She also said to him that it would make a huge difference if, every now and then, he got home five minutes earlier than he had planned. Also, if he just sent a text to say he would be five or ten minutes late, that would be OK too: at least she could adapt to that. He didn't realise the importance of this at the time.

Paul loves and respects his wife even more since she gave birth to their children. He admits that the physical relationship does change, after having watched your wife give birth. He believes that men need to take the plunge and make that effort to reconnect physically and emotionally with their wife.

Dads need to be empowered. He thinks it's important for a mother to go out for a couple of hours and leave the baby in the dad's care, with the dad being allowed to do things their own way. He believes men surprise themselves with how well they can manage when they're given the space to do it.

Barry, Age 36, Dublin

Barry doesn't remember a negative impact on his relationship with his wife after the birth of his first child, though after the second they were a lot more tired and had a lot less time for each other. They used to head out to restaurants at the weekends. 'We made a conscious decision that this wasn't going to completely change our lives. If we want to do something, we will do it, we'll just bring the child with us.' It was important for their sanity. He feels he was lucky, as he was well prepared for the changes that were coming with the arrival of their baby. He knows a lot of friends and colleagues who weren't as prepared mentally, and didn't adapt.

Simon Age 45, Dublin

The dynamic between Simon and his wife quickly changed after their first baby arrived. Suddenly his wife wasn't focused on him any more. 'Our relationship changed and I know rationally it's going to grow back to what it was, but it's going to take a number of years to grow back in that direction as the kids get bigger. There's actually a sense of bereavement, that the carefree days that we had are going to be temporarily on ice.'

When his wife needed him a lot in the first few months after the birth of their first baby, it was frustrating. 'I had to get used to the idea that she needed me so much. I was trying to balance that with the idea that our new business needed to float and not contract.' His wife wasn't able to see that he couldn't do both, and it was very difficult. He didn't say much at the time.

He remembers seeing his wife being very focused and efficient to survive those early months of motherhood. 'But then, she turned into this person who was less warm, because she was trying to be a survivor. Suddenly I was working with and for this person, instead of being in a relationship with them. It just takes the warm and fuzzy part out of the relationship.' Luckily, that warm and

fuzzy feeling did return. He feels that their relationship has deep-
ened and he has a new-found respect for his wife, as he has wit-
nessed how well she has coped with caring for both their children.

Terry, Age 40, Dublin

Terry was shocked by the effect the tiredness had on their relationship. 'My mood was black, and then naturally enough you start
taking it out on each other.' He had a great friend who could tell
him that what they were going through was completely natural.
He reassured him that this wasn't the dissolution of their relationship but actually tiredness and fatigue taking its toll. He remembers sleeping in separate beds on and off for a year and a half. 'We
would meet on the landing, fighting about whose turn it was.' He
also wasn't prepared for the impact this would have on his sex life:
they were just too exhausted. 'You stop dating, and you become
mummy and daddy. You have to make time for it.' He would advise
new mums to be compassionate and remember that there are two
people in this experience, and to try not to block the dad out.

However, he does believe that having their baby enriched their
relationship. 'I feel a connection to her that I didn't feel before we
had children, I feel that we're part of each other, completely and
utterly. It's not as exciting, but it's definitely deeper.'

Ken, Age 39, Cork

Ken has heard some dads talking about jealousy or resentment of
their baby's close relationship with their partners. 'I didn't have any
of that, but I did wonder "Where [has] my life gone?"' He and his
wife knew each other for a long time before they had children, and
he believes this helped to protect their relationship during the difficult first few months after the baby's arrival. 'I was very conscious
of my wife expecting me home at the time I said I would be home,
so I always got home on time.' They worked hard at nurturing their

relationship. 'Chocolate, alcohol, sex and comedy are just some of the things we used to keep our relationship healthy.' He was very involved in the care of his son and daughter. 'I think that most dads probably want to be involved in caring for their babies. Mums should let their husbands be involved as much as possible.'

Sex After Childbirth

Interviewees were asked about how they felt about sex after childbirth. Most of them were nervous, worrying about various things from potential pain and discomfort to how it would feel for their partners. I have compiled a list of their concerns, thoughts and realisations:

- Sex would feel different for both of them.
- Nervous that it would hurt, despite wanting to have sex.
- Just wanted to get it over with.
- One partner didn't ask if it hurt, and that bothered her. He said it didn't feel different.
- Worried that breast milk would spurt if he touches her breasts.
- Nervous that it would be different, in a bad way.
- Terrified she would damage herself; wanted to get it over with.
- First time wasn't great, but got better after that.
- Libido was high but energy was too low to have sex.
- First time having sex was more uncomfortable after caesarean than after vaginal birth.
- Worried that sex won't feel the same.

- Worried about pain from the episiotomy scar.

- Nervous that her vagina has gotten a lot bigger.

- Husband loving his wife's bigger chest and wanted sex all the time. Sometimes she just wanted a hug.

- Acceptance that she just had to do it. Terrified beforehand of pain, but it was fine.

- Worry about the pain from the stitches meant she put it off. It felt OK when they finally did have sex.

- Exhausted from breastfeeding and not comfortable with how sex fits with the role of being a mother.

- A mental block about sex, despite feeling well physically.

- Just too tired to have sex; libido was very low.

Little Gems of Advice

- Stress and tiredness relating to parenthood can have a major effect on your relationship. Don't expect too much from each other in the first few months, emotionally or physically. You are both in survival mode.

- If you find that you are snapping at each other and losing the connection you had before the baby came along, it might be good to acknowledge what's happening in your relationship, before it spirals out of control.

- Your partner may have to show strength of character when it comes to your in-laws behaving themselves (like not visiting too much/and not interfering). Consider discussing any potential issues with your in-laws before the birth.

- If there were things that annoyed or irritated you about

your partner, or vice versa, that have never been addressed, it's likely that these will become even more obvious after you have a baby. Try to sort them out before the baby arrives if you can.

- Let your partner care for the baby in his own way; your way isn't always the right way. Don't disempower him by taking over all the time if you don't like the way he is doing something. He might just end up leaving it all to you as a result.

- If you shared chores at home before the baby arrived, there is no reason why that should change just because you are at home with your baby. You are working full time caring for this baby and recovering from nine months of pregnancy and childbirth.

- Lots of people have that 'who's more tired than who' competition, along with the 'who's turn is it' competition. You're not alone.

- Whenever you can, try to do something that you used to do together as a couple, even if it's as simple as having a takeaway and a glass of wine with a movie.

- Find a babysitter.

- Encourage your partner to talk to other dads about how their relationship changed after they had children. It may help him to understand what's happening with yours.

- Try to make some time for yourself. This will, in turn, help your relationship.

- If you feel that an unequal division of labour has emerged with regards to caring for your baby, and this bothers you, try to talk about it. It can be difficult for the dad to find his role in parenting; the mother's role is often so much clearer.

- Once you emerge from the fog of early parenthood, make time for each other (e.g. organise regular date-nights) and nurture your relationship.

- Before the baby arrives, discuss what sex will be like after the birth, so that you understand each other's expectations.

- Be clear with your partner about what you need from them.

Anne's Pointers

I often see women nagging their partner about how they are doing things. Sometimes with hormones and tiredness, the smallest thing becomes a big deal: I was in a house one night and the mother criticised her partner about how he tied the nappy bag. Men can sometimes feel useless and helpless. Communicate with them. Give them lists, or specific jobs to do, and let them do them. Let them make and learn from the mistakes with the baby, as you do. For example, if they don't wind the baby well, let them deal with the consequences of a crying baby without accusing them. Don't forget to keep including your partner; maybe ask him to do the bath with the baby or to do an evening feed. They need to bond with their baby too, and do it in a different way to the mother.

Remember that your partner was there before the baby arrived, and you want him there when the baby leaves home, so this relationship is important. Try and get out together – even just for an hour – as often as you can.

9.
Routines

There are countless books on the shelves of our bookshops about how to get your baby into a routine: some are more 'hardcore' than others. On top of that, there are endless discussions online between mothers and 'experts' about the best way to get your baby into their routine, or conversely, why getting them into a routine will damage them psychologically.

In this chapter, women talk about their experience with routines and how, in some cases, it drove them crazy. Some women did have success with implementing routines, but in some cases, what worked with their first baby didn't work with their second. So is it all down to the baby? The general consensus from the interviewees is that it's rare to have success with a routine with a very young baby. Waiting until six weeks or more before starting to gently push them towards any kind of routine may be a more sensible option.

Kate, Age 38, Dublin

When my first baby was two weeks old, I remarked to my friend, who was a paediatric nurse, that my baby had done something out of the norm. My friend laughed out loud and said, "She doesn't usually do that? The norm? She's two weeks old!" My friend explained that the baby doesn't have a 'usually'; she doesn't have a norm that she will change over and over and over again, especially in these early weeks. Now, looking back, I realise that she was right. I thought, like many new mothers, that I could have some sense of control. I wish I had spent more time holding and loving my baby, following her lead on sleep and feeding, instead of trying to push her into a routine that she was never going to go into at a few weeks of age.

With my second baby, I was more relaxed about routines, although I did find myself trying to stretch my baby between feeds when he was eight weeks old. I started to panic about breastfeeding him too often, until a breastfeeding counsellor at a local breastfeeding group asked me what was wrong with him feeding a bit more often during the day, if night-times were going OK. She was dead right. Then I just went with whatever he needed, trusting that he would know when he needed to eat and sleep. Life has felt a lot calmer and less stressful that way. You can't make a baby go to sleep if they don't want to sleep. I continued this approach into his fifth month, and he gradually sorted out his own routine.

Deborah, Age 37, Dublin

Some good advice that Deborah received in the early months was that whatever stage life was at with this new baby, it wasn't going to be like that forever – that phases come and go. She remembers asking the advice of another mother with regards to getting her baby to understand the difference between night and day. Her friend advised her to bring the baby upstairs at 7 PM every night and to be there with the baby quietly, in dimmed lighting, to get her used to the fact that this was wind-down time. One of her initial reactions was to worry about the effect this would have on her relationship, as she wouldn't get to see her husband at all and wasn't going to do it. Her friend assured her that this was only going to be for a few weeks. At the time it felt like she was giving up her evenings with her husband forever.

Jenny, Age 35, Dublin

Jenny resisted routine in the early days. However, she remembers that in the first few weeks, in the evenings when her husband came home and dinner was being prepared, the baby got quite irritable and it all felt a bit manic. She realises now that when they focused on making that part of the day a calm time and started cluster-feeding (which also helped with sleeping), things got a lot better.

Kerry, Age 37, Dublin

Before she even had her baby, a woman Kerry used to meet kept trying to convert her to the sleeping routines of a particular baby 'expert'. 'It was like her mission to convert me. I read one page and then thought, she's a complete lunatic and she would never suit me anyway, because of all those regimented lists.'

Elaine, Age 29, Dublin

Elaine wanted routine with her baby. After about sixteen weeks, her baby got into her own routine, and she just went with it. Even after two years, she is happy in her night time routine as it's how it's always been for her. She doesn't believe you can get a baby into a routine at three or four weeks. 'You can't do it with a new baby, and don't try; it's not going to work.'

Ella, Age 45, Dublin

Ella found it very hard not to have control in the early weeks. 'I wanted to have a sense of achievement, and if this was what my job was, I wanted to do it right. Then you get a little routine going, and in a couple of days or weeks that would go completely because the baby was changing constantly.' Her biggest frustration was not being able to stick to the schedule she had created for herself and her baby. 'I had to get out for a walk at one o'clock. Where was I going? I was setting ridiculous small daily goals and tasks so I felt like I was achieving, doing a good job and being supermum. I was failing at everything in the beginning because I was trying to achieve things.' Her mum wisely advised her to stop making lists, telling her that she wasn't going to a meeting, she was raising a baby. As soon as she got her head around that things became much easier.

Fionnuala, Age 40, Dublin

Fionnuala felt she was obsessed with her son's sleeping routine, how much her son slept, or how long he had slept for. She now wishes she had just watched him to see what his routine was. She remembers reading a book about routines early on, and when the book said he needed a lunch time feed, she fed him at 12.50 and felt she had failed as it wasn't lunchtime yet. 'I still do it about his sleeping. Her son is now two years old.'

Suzy, Age 36, Dublin

Suzy followed a very strict routine from quite early on with her baby. She is glad that she did it, but she became obsessed with sleep and routine.

Andrea, Age 38, Dublin

Andrea had prepared a lot for the birth of her first baby. She had read books promoting strict routines as well as those promoting a more relaxed approach, and found her own balance somewhere in the middle. From about seven weeks she started to gently push her baby towards a sleeping and feeding routine, and by eleven weeks she had cracked it and her baby was sleeping really well.

Once Andrea got her daughter in to a routine, she remembers being terrified that if she changed anything, the whole thing would fall apart. If she was late with a scheduled feed, she started thinking that it would have a knock-on effect and her whole life would be ruined, never mind her day. Her second baby nearly broke her. 'He wasn't interested in sleeping.' She tried everything. He was seven months old before she got him sleeping through to 5 AM. All babies are different.

Isobel, Age 39, Dublin

Isobel breastfed her babies. She had many people around her who were purists, demand-feeding their babies and being anti-routine. Looking back, she feels that she should have tried to get her babies into a routine after the first few weeks, despite the fact that she was breastfeeding. She feels that if she could have got them into a routine, she could have looked after herself and her mental health more than she did.

Laoise, Age 37, Dublin

In the first few weeks after the birth of her son, Laoise was 'mental with routines'. People used to ask her when he had fed or slept, so she felt like she should know. She started to write down everything about his feeds and sleeps. 'I thought, I'll watch his patterns for a while, and he will start to form a pattern. I think he was fourteen months old when he started to have a pattern.'

She felt stressed out when she was feeding on demand and wondered whether she would she ever get him into a routine. Her midwife told her not to bother, but she liked to know what might happen at certain times of the day. The GP told her to give it six weeks and then to start thinking about a routine.

At about three months her son started getting in to a very loose routine. She could never get him to sleep. 'I found that really stressful because I thought I was failing. I was getting stressed because I was sure that if I did things differently during the day, he would sleep at night.'

Her friend gave her great advice in telling her to lower her expectations, which is what she did on her second child. She felt it really helped as she didn't stress as much about sleep and routines.'

Barbara, Age 32, Dublin

Barbara had read all the books and was convinced by them that her twin boys would go into a routine from only a few weeks old. She tried again and again to put them into a routine but failed in these early weeks. She now feels that 'The first three months is a special time. Ignore what the books say; it's really hard to put your baby into a routine.' She thinks that if your baby is falling into his or her own natural routine, you should go with it. In the first three months, she advises not meeting people for coffee in every spare moment. 'You have to accept that you're in a bubble for that first three months. You have to take care of you, your relationship and your baby and just be in the bubble. You'll never get this chance again to be in that new-family phase.'

Little Gems of Advice

- People lie. Don't always believe what people tell you about how well their babies are sleeping. For some reason, some new parents do this. Not everyone is able to be honest about how hard they are finding it.

- Just because one mum has had a negative experience with regards to change in routine at various developmental stages, doesn't mean you will. Your baby is different to every other baby.

- If you get your baby into a routine, don't be surprised when the routine changes soon afterwards. Babies' needs change all the time, so their routine will too.

- In those early weeks, follow your baby's lead when it comes to sleeping and feeding. It's very difficult to push them into a routine before six to eight weeks. Even then, it can cause more stress for both you and your baby.

- Sticking to a very rigid routine can lead to disappointment and frustration when your baby 'doesn't play ball'.

- Many mothers said that the eight-to-twelve week mark is when a baby can start being gently pushed in to a routine.

- If imposing a routine feels wrong, just go with the baby's lead. Some parents find routines stressful and restrictive. It depends on your personality. Some parents crave routine, as do some babies.

Anne's Pointers

When routine goes awry during the day don't panic. Take each day as a new day and a new start.

10.
Tiredness

Looking back at my experience as a first-time mum, tiredness was my arch-enemy. It comes up in almost every conversation about childbirth and those early months of motherhood. Tiredness affects everyone differently, from irritability, paranoia and anxiety to physical symptoms of nausea, dizziness and headaches. Almost every mother I interviewed could not stress enough the importance of grabbing any opportunity to sleep or rest when it comes along. Go to bed. When you are tired, the smallest of problems becomes insurmountable, and decisions that were once easy to make become impossible.

Kate, Age 38, Dublin

I had never experienced tiredness quite like this. I didn't realise at the time that this was what had affected me most. Apart from making me irritable and unreasonable, tiredness made me a bit paranoid and unable to make the most basic decisions. I never agreed with the advice to sleep when the baby sleeps, but now I realise that it makes sense.

At the time, I thought I had to keep the house relatively tidy and cook meals, and wash clothes. Why didn't I ask for more help? Why didn't I just go to bed? I was too hung up on being a good hostess, an efficient and competent homemaker, a caring partner and the perfect mother. Wasn't I the fool.

After my second baby, my husband and I made sleep a priority. The guest room, and ear plugs, were used most nights for the first five or six months. Instead of opting for private maternity care, we used the money to pay for a night nurse for a few nights, as well as regular home help. This helped to get us through the really sleep-deprived times. Apart from one or two bad days, I can't compare the tiredness this time round with the first time. That's down to the help we got, and the fact that we made sleep our priority.

Deirdre, Age 40, Dublin

Deirdre experienced tiredness as much as any new mother. 'It means you can't deal with everyday issues; everything gets blown out of proportion. You can cope with anything if you get your sleep.' She and her husband ended up taking one night each 'on duty', so at least they always knew that they would have a full night's sleep the next night. 'I did let the house go to rack and ruin. I was willing to let things go to get more sleep. To me, getting your sleep is the biggest thing to help you deal with everything else.'

Isobel, Age 39, Dublin

Isobel recommends that, if possible, anyone who is bringing a new baby home should try to get a cleaner in for a few hours a week. This, along with stocking up the freezer with healthy meals in advance, will help with the tiredness, as you will need the time and the energy for other things.

On her first baby, she remembers the exhaustion of the constant feeding and changing. She remembers one night, crazy with tiredness, as her baby wouldn't settle, saying to her husband, 'Take her off me or I'm going to f*** her against the wall.' She feels that if you get to that stage of tiredness, you should get someone to spend one or two nights in your home, looking after the baby, so that you can get some sleep.

Sinead, Age 37, Cork

Sinead got used to the tiredness and started to be able to function extremely well with only four hours' sleep. 'Don't think it's the end of your life and your life will always be like this, because it does change.' She feels that even if you find it difficult to fall asleep for short naps during the day, try to get some quiet time to clear your head. 'After you've had a baby, you never switch off. Even when you're asleep, you have one ear open in case they cry for you.' If someone else can take the baby and let you have a shower or read a book, it helps a lot. That being said, she remembers her mum offering to take the baby so that she could leave the house, but she didn't want to leave him; she felt that she would be abandoning him if she left.

Marie, Age 49, Dublin

For Marie, the tiredness in the early weeks of motherhood reduced her day-to-day experience to something like a struggle to survive. 'I need my sleep. I can remember feeling a bit like there was no difference between day and night, and it all became a blur. That was overwhelming.' She doesn't know how she would have coped if her husband hadn't taken care of all the household chores for them.

She believes that new mothers have to 'sleep at every opportunity rather than thinking that anything else could be a priority other than you and the baby. You are the most precious two things in this world at this time, and these moments won't come again. All they need is you, and all you need is them.' Even if you don't sleep, she would encourage any new mother to rest and accept all help that is offered.

Ruth, Age 36, Kildare

Ruth remembers well the tiredness with her first baby: it reduced her to tears. 'You don't even have the energy to make a sandwich, you're so tired.' Even when her baby slept, she couldn't sleep, as she was worried about his breathing. 'You can't relax because you're so worried about them.' She found it very hard to relax, on all three of her babies. 'One benefit of breastfeeding is that you actually have to physically sit down and relax to feed the baby.' Her advice to any new mother would be that even if you're not sleeping, at least try to rest and not run around the house cleaning.

Jenny, Age 35, Dublin

Jenny was fortunate to have a baby that slept really well from quite early on. She didn't have the experience of extreme tiredness that many mothers report. Of the tiredness that she did experience, she said, 'You can't think properly, you can't function properly, and you're learning this thing that's so new, but you're learning in a way that you haven't before. Put tiredness into that mix, and it can become a bit emotional.'

Mary, Age 32, Tipperary

Mary found that she did really well in the first few weeks, as she just told herself to get on with it and 'suck it up', despite having to-do all the night-feeds at the beginning because she was breastfeed-ing. However, after a few weeks she felt that it got more difficult. 'I found myself getting a bit low sometimes' but it was all worth it and it improved with time. People told her to sleep when the baby slept, but she found it difficult to ignore housework. 'I just wasn't good at going to sleep when she was sleeping. I know I should do that the next time.' She remembers at about four to six weeks thinking that she felt like she was getting a bit depressed. 'I felt like I never got outside this door because I was up all night, and getting up late . . . One night was running in to the next.' The first six weeks are still quite hazy for her, but after that things did change for the better.

Laoise, Age 37, Dublin

Laoise dealt quite well with the tiredness in the first two months after her first baby was born. However, after that first two months she started to feel very slow mentally; she couldn't even think about shopping lists for dinner. 'It affected my ability to do everything; things took me forever; I was a dimwit.' She believes that she shouldn't have picked her baby up to feed him at every turn, but instead should have left him to settle himself a little. 'I cannot listen to children crying, but we ultimately did have to leave him cry it out after six months. If we had let a little bit of crying happen earlier, maybe after the three-month mark, it wouldn't have got to such a crisis point at a later stage.'

Rebecca, Age 41, Kilkenny

Rebecca remembers that the tiredness really muddled her brain 'You're just surviving, just getting through one half of the day to the next.' She found it hard to leave the washing and housework so that she could sleep, even though she knew it made sense. 'It sounds easy, but it's not . . . You just feel like you're failing in some way.' She doesn't find it easy to ask for help. She believes that women are often so ingrained in their roles in the home that they sometimes don't ask for help with things like cooking and housework. 'Partners are much more available than we give them credit for. If they ask you can they get you a cup of tea, a glass of water or a sandwich, say "Yes please!"'

Barbara, Age 32, Dublin

For Barbara and her husband, the tiredness of having newborn twin babies meant that their minds were completely muddled, making them unable to see the obvious solutions to problems. 'When we took them home, every night for four nights, they were happy when they were in our arms, and then we put them down, and five minutes later, just as they were going to sleep, they were screaming crying.' Her husband eventually, after four days and nights of no sleep, realised that the babies were simply too cold. They just hadn't thought that that might be a problem.

For her, tiredness affected her like the worst hangover ever, along with a pounding headache. She felt like vomiting, and her whole body hurt from the total exhaustion.

Emma, Age 44, Kildare

She would advise a new mother: 'Take all the help you can get. If anyone offers to do anything, take it. You'll be so tired.' The best present Emma ever received was a lasagne from her sister and brother in-law, delivered to the door. She copes fairly well without sleep, but only because she has to. In the early days with a new baby, 'You would be completely stupid. You don't know where you are.' She used to try to go upstairs and sleep with her new baby, but that's not proper sleep, she says. You need someone to come and mind the baby. 'Somebody to come in and do laundry and do dinners would be great. Then you could enjoy your baby.'

Roisín, Age 38, Dublin

Roisín normally copes quite well without sleep. 'I think it helped a lot, I've always been someone who stores sleep. I didn't have a hard time with sleep with my first baby either.' She had her second child very quickly after her first. 'The first time I realised what sleep deprivation felt like was just before my eldest daughter's fifth birthday. Neither of the girls were sleeping properly, and hadn't been for a couple of weeks.' She realised then what it must have been like for her friends who experienced awful tiredness after having their babies.

Deborah, Age 37, Dublin

Deborah believes that getting back to yoga classes after seven weeks was a lifeline. She went to very gentle classes and it helped her to be in better form. She believes that, for her, gentle exercise, and the time it gave her to herself, was a real help with regards to tiredness and her overall happiness.

Kerry, Age 37, Dublin

Kerry would describe herself as 'not very practical'. She didn't read baby books or instruction manuals for equipment before the baby was born. She was nearly crying from tiredness. She couldn't remember basic things like when she had fed her baby or how the straps on the pram worked. Everything seemed to be a huge challenge. The 'sleep when the baby sleeps' advice didn't resonate with her at all when she had her baby. In retrospect, she feels it might have been the best piece of advice she was given. 'I quickly realised how important sleep was, and how much I need it.'

Elaine, Age 29, Dublin

'I wish I had slept a bit more, when the baby was asleep. I was so wound up when the house was untidy.' She would advise anyone having a baby, if they can, to get in a cleaner or someone to do the basic tidying up and cooking.

Caroline, Age 35, Dublin

Caroline did pay attention to the 'sleep when the baby sleeps' advice that she got, and that helped to cope with the tiredness. She had a co-sleeper bed with her second baby, and although he may have woken more than her first, it was so easy to just pull him into the bed and feed him. She would advise any new mum not to worry about cleaning the house, going out and meeting people or visitors. 'Go up and sleep with your baby; cancel visitors.' Her yoga teacher advised her to stay in her pyjamas for two weeks, that people wouldn't expect anything of her then.

Alison, Age 38, Kildare/San Francisco

Alison's mother stayed with friends nearby. She used to take the baby at 6 AM for a couple of hours so that Alison and her partner could sleep.

Alison thinks that saved her. 'If I got three hours of uninterrupted sleep, I could get through the day.'

Astrid, Age 39, Germany/Dublin

Astrid is usually pretty good surviving on little sleep, but like most women found the first two weeks very tiring. 'I remember that I was out and about, meeting friends and doing things, not like I would do now, but still.' She remembers, though, that breastfeeding did make her very tired some days. 'With both kids, I would often just fall asleep with them at 8 PM. I did that for a long time, until I stopped feeding them at over a year old.'

Megan, Age 40, Dublin

Megan would normally have managed with tiredness very well, as she seemed to have an energy reserve to tap into. 'After having my son, I found I had no reserve. It's like jet lag . . . You need to nap. I said "yes" to every bit of help that was offered to me.' She slept when her baby slept. 'You can't plough through that kind of tiredness; your body is recovering from childbirth.'

Sarah, Age 37, Cork/London

After she was born, Sarah's second baby was in the hospital's Special Care Baby Unit for more than ten days. Sarah stayed at the hospital and had to express every four hours, as her baby was being tube-fed. It was a long process, with all the sterilisation that was involved. Sarah could only have very short stretches of sleep, and of course the worry didn't help. 'I wasn't starting from a very good point – exhausted before you leave the hospital.' Sarah usually copes really well with tiredness and her attitude is to get up and get on with it. When she was tired, she felt 'constantly grumpy and cranky and emotional.'

Her husband was very supportive and would help wherever he could, but with breastfeeding she was always the one up at night, and getting up every couple of hours did wear her down. She felt that sometimes he didn't really understand how tiring it was. 'He used to say he was busy all day and it's not like he had time to himself, but I was jealous of him getting on the train in the morning for his commute, where he had half an hour of headspace. I remember being very emotional, and I think a lot of that is down to tiredness. If you have a couple of good night sleep the whole world looks better.'

Rachel, Age 41, Dublin

Rachel's partner was not working during her maternity leave, so they were both at home. 'If I went for a nap, he would take her up. It was a very languid time.' All she had to do was feed her, as she had that support at home, and she felt like it was just the three of them in a lovely bubble. 'I didn't think that I could have children, so she was this gift. She was a good baby, so that has to have helped.' She hadn't read many baby books beforehand. 'It was one of the only things I had planned . . . getting sleep, not responding to every mooch and not disturbing her sleep, no matter how tempted you might be to pick her up.'

Yvonne, Age 40, Dublin

On her third baby, Yvonne felt her age and found the night-feeds so much more difficult than with her previous children. 'My husband was eleven years older than me, and he was getting up at 6.30 AM for work and I was complaining. I wasn't even in work, but

I had to get up for my other daughter. I found that really, really tough. I couldn't do the "sleep when the baby sleeps" because my daughter was there too.'

'I was very cranky, very snappy. It was like you had no blood in your body. It was very difficult to get through the day; you'd be watching the clock waiting for night-time.' Her husband did the last night-feed while she was in bed and she would do the middle-of-the-night feed, and that helped them to cope. 'You have to do a rota to decide who's doing what.'

Kathleen, Age 38, Donegal

Kathleen thinks that the tiredness you experience after childbirth is different to other tiredness. 'You're so tired, but you have forgotten the fact that you're tired, and you think there has to be something else wrong with you other than the fact that you're absolutely exhausted. There's no recovery from the tiredness, and then a little bit of low-level panic sets in, as you think you're never going to get a rest again. You get up every day and it's about survival. When are they going to sleep? How am I going to get through this? What's next?'

She would advise any new mother to stay out of hospital if it's not an environment that is conducive to sleep. If you do stay in hospital, bring an eye-mask and earplugs. If someone offers to take your baby to give you a break, let them do it. 'You are going to be exhausted after the birth, but try not to be exhausted because you stayed up for two nights beforehand cleaning the house.'

In the weeks after the birth, she was not worried as much about the baby as she was about her sleep. She knew the baby would be fine. 'You do really need to look after yourself, even if that means giving the baby away to someone for twenty-four hours. I think a night nurse is a great idea. They bring the baby to you to be fed and take the baby away to be changed, so that all you do is feed them and then you go back to sleep.' She says that, looking back at the early weeks with her first baby, she should have given the baby to someone to take out of the house so that she could have slept. 'I had this sense that I had to look after her.'

Michelle, Age 30, Dublin

Michelle read lots of books on babies and sleep. 'Nobody tells you that your baby might cry hysterically, to the point where they are shaking and you are afraid they are going to have an aneurysm.' The first two or three months weren't too bad for them, but by the four-month mark things had changed. Her baby's sleep became very disrupted. Michelle and her husband had no idea why. They were very sleep-deprived. When he had to get up on occasion, Michelle would feel guilty. On the other hand, once she had been up a few times during the night, ahead of another full day minding the baby, she stopped caring if her husband was having to get up at night too. 'For whatever reason, I don't think people really see looking after a kid as a "real job". I find it really annoying when people keep asking me when I'm going back to work: this is the most important job I've ever had.'

Anna, Age 37, Dublin

Anna found that the tiredness of becoming a mum made her really emotional. 'I would dissolve into tears, be quite paranoid. You're second-guessing everything you're doing. There were times when I was so tired, if I didn't lie down I would actually fall down ... when it was verging on delirium.' One thing that she wishes she hadn't done in the first few weeks was obsess about getting the baby down into the cot after she fell asleep in Anna's arms. When they did this, she would wake up screaming, as she had reflux and needed to be upright after being fed. However, with her second baby she didn't want to make the same mistake, and kept her baby in the bed with her. 'Everybody kept telling me "You can't bring her into the bed", but for the first six weeks that child shouldn't have been anywhere else but in my arms.'

Her advice for a new mother would be for the parents to sleep in separate rooms in the early days, so that at least one parent is sleeping. Also, if possible, new parents should get a cleaner in, or at least get help at home.

Anna always thought that her baby sleeping through the night meant that the baby would sleep for twelve hours. 'I thought they would do that from about six weeks. When everybody talked to me about their baby sleeping through the night, they were lying!'

Gemma, Age 40, Dublin

Gemma hadn't realised how exhausted she was until several months after her first baby was born. She had never experienced tiredness like that before. 'It felt fuzzy, a haze, like your body wasn't your own and your mind was working on autopilot. I was definitely very irritable.' She thinks the only way to be less tired is to sleep when the baby sleeps, get people to bring dinners, have a shower every day to help yourself wake up, and get your partner to do the 11 PM feed, with an expressed bottle or a bottle of formula. 'One of the nicest presents we got was a few stews that appeared at our front door.'

Ella, Age 45, Dublin

Ella thought she wasn't that tired in the first two weeks and felt like she was doing OK. Her baby was feeding every twenty minutes. 'I remember looking out the window thinking I must tell my husband to sort out those cockroaches. I was awake but my mind wanted to be asleep: there were no cockroaches. It's like that tiredness when you've been drinking all night and you've gone to work the next day. You can't go to bed and there are moments when your mind wants to switch off . . . That's the kind of feeling I had.' She realised then that she was truly exhausted.

When the baby was asleep, she struggled with the advice to sleep when they are sleeping. 'It didn't work for me. If I'm going to be in the house, it can't be a complete mess, because that was the one thing that was likely to make me depressed.'

Fionnuala, Age 40, Dublin

When Fionnuala came down from the initial high of her baby arriving, she felt she lacked strategies for sleeping, such as how to feed the baby while lying on her side. 'I should have had no visitors and stayed in bed, morning till night.' She feels she needed to have someone there checking she was OK and reminding her to go back to bed.

There was a long time during which her son didn't sleep in the evenings, and got up late in the morning. 'I fought that for so long and tried to make him into one of those children who would go to bed early, and he just would not. This idea of having your evenings back: some people get them, but loads don't, and we were one of those couples who didn't.'

Suzy, Age 36, Dublin

Suzy would have managed on very little sleep before she became a mother but still found the tiredness difficult. 'There is a reason that they use sleep deprivation as a method of torture . . . It totally works.'

Emma, Age 33, Dublin

Emma was very fortunate, as they had a lot of support both from her mother and her mother-in-law. She and her husband were able to take time off early on, including a three-day holiday in the sun without the baby, when her firstborn was ten weeks old. 'With one baby it was like a little fairy tale, having the two mams living near us.' All this support really helped them to cope with those first few months of parenthood.

Heather, Age 39, Dublin

One of the hardest things in the early months of motherhood for Heather was realising what lack of sleep means. 'There's no end to it, no break, no relief.' Her baby fed around the clock, up to an hour on each breast. It was like an endless cycle. After three weeks she thought she couldn't continue, as it was so relentless and tiring. She believes that the hormones produced during breastfeeding keep you going during the sleepless nights. She was surviving on three or four hours a night, which she found amazing. 'There were times when I thought, I'm not going to drive the car today, it's too dangerous.' She expressed a bottle of milk so that her husband would do one of the feeds, in order to give her a few hours' sleep in the evenings. Their son wasn't a great sleeper and they ended up doing sleep training with him at eight months, but Heather wishes she had done it earlier, at about six months.

Patricia, Age 35, Dublin

Patricia was lucky that her first son slept very well from six weeks. She experienced awful tiredness up to then. It used to annoy her when people said 'sleep when the baby sleeps' but she now realises what they actually mean is that if you can pick up a bit of sleep during the day, do it. 'If your neighbour comes in and says, "Will I take the baby for a walk for an hour?" you say "Yes please. Thank you very much."' Many women seem to find it difficult to hand their first baby over in this way. She remembers anxiously standing at the window after an hour and ten minutes when her neighbour had brought the baby for an hour's walk, awaiting their return.

Patricia would advise any new mother not to underestimate how refreshed you can feel even after just forty-five minutes' sleep. Take it when you can.

Julianne, Age 39, Tipperary

Julianne is still tired, even though her second baby is eleven months old. 'I don't know how to describe it. At times it's all-consuming, and all you want to do is sleep for another half an hour.' She still has a nap any time she gets a chance. Even though it's a bit boring, and everyone says it, she does recommend that you sleep when the baby sleeps. 'On your first, you can do it. You don't believe how easy it is with one, until you have two. No matter how much my sister told me, I wouldn't believe her.'

Andrea, Age 38, Dublin

Andrea worked in a high-stress job where she had to work all-nighters. 'I knew I could physically do it. I have literally been trained to go without sleep for long periods of time.' She approached the early months of motherhood like a work project. 'I actually coped with it very well.' She had worked as a nanny and au pair for young babies in the past, so she had no preconceptions that this was going to be easy. 'Going into it like that, I was mentally prepared for my first baby.' It helped that her first baby was a fairly good sleeper.

Her second baby nearly broke her. He had no interest in sleeping or routines. I got really, really depressed with him, I just felt like I couldn't do it. As it was second time round I was exhausted. I had no reserves, so I couldn't do the "project" thing.

In retrospect, she feels that she should have gone to bed more. She and her husband now take turns to get up if their children wake, and she wears earplugs, because otherwise she knows she will be the one who will wake and get up to comfort them. When that happens, she finds herself asking ' "Why the hell am I doing this? Why isn't he getting up? It's his turn." But he feels completely disempowered because I haven't even given him the chance to do it. It's the letting go of control.'

Helena, Age 33, Dublin

Helena found that the tiredness of early motherhood made her feel quite dizzy sometimes. She remembers going to a clinic for injections for her baby and 'they were asking me what my name was. I had to think hard about my name and the date of birth of the baby.' She found the simplest things so hard to do, and found it really hard to concentrate on anything. 'Leaving the clinic I had to lie down: I thought I was going to collapse.'

The Dad's Point of View

Simon, Age 45, Dublin

In the early months, Simon found that the tiredness restricted his ability to think strategically in work, to see the bigger picture. 'I end up just constricting down to day-to-day functionality.'

Barry, Age 36, Dublin

Barry doesn't remember major tiredness in the early months. His wife was breastfeeding so he didn't have to get up at night to feed the baby. 'I did wake a lot, and looking back I think why didn't I just sleep in the spare room?'

He thinks that if he had been up feeding his baby in the middle of the night, it would have been difficult to get up and go to work. 'For a man to try to explain that to a woman who has just had a baby . . . you're on dangerous ground there! Mothers need to understand that their life is totally consumed by the baby, and rightly so, but the rest of the world goes on and doesn't really care, including the guy who's paying your husband.' Work was difficult for him at the time, so it was lovely to come home to his wife and new baby.

Terry, Age 40, Dublin

Terry feels that nobody prepares you properly for the tiredness that follows the birth of your child. 'I think that it's completely sugar-coated, and parents don't want to let you know that you're in for a tough, tough ride. The tiredness nearly killed us.'

He felt like he was cracking up, unable to function properly, going in to work in ribbons. He felt he was like having an out-of-body experience. 'You're in your own body but someone has taken over your mind. You're brainwashed by fatigue . . . walking around like a zombie.'

If he had a big day at work, he would stay at a friend's house to ensure he got some sleep. 'If you took away the tiredness, I would say that this is just magical.' He thinks people need to make it a priority to obtain whatever help is necessary to ensure they can get sufficient sleep.

Ken, Age 39, Cork

Ken's first baby was not a good sleeper. They had a really tough time in the early months. His wife opted for co-sleeping. 'I should have slept in the spare room. I didn't. My advice for dads is: don't be a martyr, go and sleep in the spare room one or two nights a week.'

Looking back, he realises that he should have felt less guilty and taken more time to sleep. 'It's hard to avoid the guilt though, but there's no point in two people not getting any sleep. A few nights' proper sleep does wonders for you both, so share the suffering!'

Little Gems of Advice

- Although it may not seem feasible when the housework is calling or visitors are arriving, try to sleep when your baby sleeps. If you can't sleep, then try to rest when they are asleep. It's a piece of advice that most of the intervieees regret not following. Try to get some help at night -time. If someone you trust is willing to look after the baby in your home for a night (even if they wake you to feed the baby), it means you can sleep more deeply knowing that someone else has their ear out for the baby.

- Don't underestimate the physical effect of tiredness. Many people interviewed felt sick, and dizzy, and had headaches from exhaustion. Make sure you get reassurance from your GP too, if any of these things are ongoing.

- Ask for help for the simple things like cooking meals and tidying the house, so that you can go to bed. Don't try to be the perfect hostess and partner, as well as the perfect mother.

- Try to put some money away during the pregnancy to put towards paying someone to help at home in the early weeks after the baby has arrived. Night nurses can help you get a full night's sleep when you really need it. If you can get a family member or a friend to help, all the better.

- If you have a voice in your head telling you that you are the one who must look after the baby all the time, remember that it's OK for someone to take the baby for a little while to give you a break. It doesn't mean that you're failing your baby.

- Look at the option of sleeping in a separate room to your

partner for the first two or three months, even if just for a few nights a week. If one of you gets a full night's sleep, it will be easier. There is no point in you both being exhausted.

- Stock your freezer with healthy dinners so you and your partner don't have to cook as frequently.

- Consider a sensor-pad mat to keep under your baby: the reassurance it provides could help you sleep more deeply, by ensuring you don't react to every snort and shuffle.

- If you find yourself despairing due to tiredness, feeling that you can't do it, or that this is your life forever, know that it will change. This is a temporary phase of your life with your new baby.

- Gentle physical activity like yoga or a short walk can help with tiredness and give you some headspace too.

- Sometimes, you're so tired you think there has to be something else physical or psychologically wrong with you other than tiredness. It may be just tiredness.

- If you don't sleep well in hospitals, make sure you bring your earplugs and an eye-mask.

- If people want to help, apart from minding your baby, suggest a home-cooked meal delivered to the door.

- If your partner is on duty to tend to the baby during the night, let them do this. Wear ear-plugs so you don't hear the baby. Make the most of the chance to grab some uninterrupted sleep.

Anne's Pointers

Tiredness is synonymous with a new baby. Don't try to be the perfect mother and perfect partner. Be kind to yourself; accept help; make sure you eat properly: a poor diet will only reduce your energy levels further. Consider getting your partner to do the last evening feed so that you can go to bed early. Work it out so that you get a run of six hours sleep, and it will make the next day an easier day.

If I had a euro for every time I was asked when the baby was going to sleep through the night, I would be a rich woman. I don't ever give specifics as every baby is different, and so many different things can affect sleeping. What I do say is that as you move forward the amount they sleep will increase, and time between feeds will stretch at night.

Resources and Useful Contacts

General Support for New Parents

Cuidiú: Education and Support for Parenthood – cuidiu-ict.ie

Many people recommended this organisation as a great support for parents. Their aim is to support parents through pregnancy, child-birth and breastfeeding. They have various websites, including Guide to Maternity Services in Ireland (bump2babe.ie) and Cuidiu ante-natal classes (antenatalireland.ie).

Rollercoaster – rollercoaster.ie

This website is a popular pregnancy and parenting website with useful forums for asking questions about pregnancy, childbirth and your baby. Also it's where I found the mums who live near me, and we formed our own mother baby group.

Parentline – parentline.ie

An organisation that provides support, guidance and information on all aspects of being a parent.

Postnatal Depression Support

PND Ireland – pnd.ie

A website and support group dedicated to postnatal depression.

AWARE – aware.ie

This organisation provides information, education and support relating to all types of depression.

Nurture – nurturepnd.org

An Irish charity offering affordable professional counselling and supports surrounding pregnancy and childbirth, mental health, and emotional well-being to women, their partners and families.

Talk to your GP if you think you might have postnatal depression.

Breastfeeding Support

Cuidiú: Education and Support for Parenthood – cuidiu-ict.ie

Many people recommended this organisation as a great support for parents. Their aim is to support parents through pregnancy, childbirth and breastfeeding.

Kelly Mom – kellymom.com

Lots of interviewees use this website. It has excellent detailed advice about breastfeeding.

HSE – breastfeeding.ie

A good source of local contacts and some nice bits of advice from other mums in video format.

La Lèche League – lalecheleagueireland.com

Access to local groups and breastfeeding information.